TESTES AND OVARIES - FUNCTIONAL AND CLINICAL DIFFERENCES AND SIMILARITIES

Edited by **Atef M. Darwish**

Testes and Ovaries - Functional and Clinical Differences and Similarities
http://dx.doi.org/10.5772/65984
Edited by Atef M. Darwish

Contributors

Alice Ioana Albu, Dragos Albu, Chantal Amisi, Mputu Lobota, Mboloko Esimo, Paolo Pozzilli, Zhengchao Wang, Fan Wang, Zonghao Tang, Atef M.M. Darwish, Roger Hart, Fiona Langdon, Jenni Pontre

Published by InTech

Janeza Trdine 9, 51000 Rijeka, Croatia

Publishing Process Manager Mirena Calmic
Technical Editor SPi Global
Cover InTech Design team

First published January, 2018
Printed in Croatia
Legal deposit, Croatia: National and University Library in Zagreb

Additional hard copies can be obtained from orders@intechopen.com

Testes and Ovaries - Functional and Clinical Differences and Similarities, Edited by Atef M. Darwish
p. cm.
Print ISBN 978-953-51-3689-7
Online ISBN 978-953-51-3690-3

For EU product safety concerns:
IN TECH d.o.o., Prolaz Marije Krucifikse Kozulić 3, 51000 Rijeka, Croatia,
info@intechopen.com or visit our website at intechopen.com.

Meet the editor

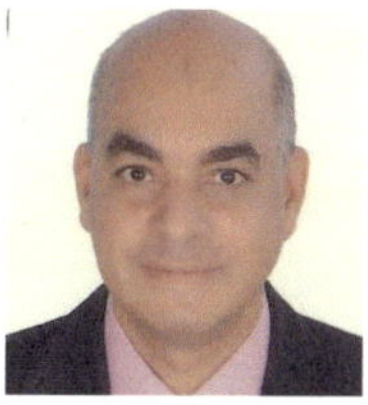

Prof. Atef M. Darwish received his MD degree from Ulm University, Ulm, Germany, and Assiut University, Assiut, Egypt, in 1994 and received his PhD degree from Utrecht University, the Netherlands, in 2009. He joined the Department of Obstetrics and Gynecology at the University of Assiut in 1986 where he was promoted first to associate professor in 2000 and then to professor in 2005. His clinical interests have mainly focused on minimally invasive gynecologic surgery as well as innovative reproductive medicine and surgery. He delivered lectures on reproductive medicine throughout the USA and Europe. His research interests have mainly focused on reproductive surgery, gynecologic endoscopy, early cervical cancer detection, and infertility. He published some innovative procedures in the field of hysteroscopic, laparoscopic, colposcopic, and minimal access surgeries in addition to drug therapy of hyperprolactinemia. He organized many training courses and delivered more than 100 lectures in different fields of obstetrics and gynecology. He is a moderator and a trainer of gynecologic endoscopy in many associations. Since 1995, he has received congress prizes and awards for his work in the field of reproductive medicine. He successfully mentored tens of master and MD degree theses and has collaborated with many other professors. He has authored over 75 scientific articles and 8 international books. He has been serving as the editor in chief and as the editorial board member of 10 leading international journals. Currently, he is involved in the clinical teaching supported by evidence-based obstetrics and gynecology and scholarly activity for the students of the University of Assiut, Egypt, in addition to working as a consultant in three hospitals.

Contents

Preface

I feel privileged to introduce this book titled ***Testes and Ovaries - Functional and Clinical Differences and Similarities.*** Its idea is unique as it is supposed to focus the attention of all scientists interested in reproduction to the idea that both sexes may have some embryological, anatomical, endocrinological, and functional differences and similarities. Testes and ovaries are an endpoint of fetal development, and the sameness of these organs is a curious fact, which makes the human anatomy more interesting compared to any other species. In order to acquire a better understanding of the genital tract in both males and females, we should primarily understand what sets them apart and what is surprisingly similar in their anatomy and their function.

The ideal clinical implication of ***Testes and Ovaries - Functional and Clinical Differences and Similarities*** concept is infertility. Both gynecologists and andrologists should have basic knowledge about both sexes during investigating and treating a couple's infertility. They should collaborate as a single team during the decision-making process and each case should be treated individually. These concepts and more will be found in a separate chapter (Chapter 1). In this chapter, both gynecologists and andrologists will find important updated information that is very helpful during the decision-making process regarding the infertility.

Since age is the most important independent factor for fertility, studies demonstrated that an increased female age and, to a lesser extent, male age could have a negative impact on fertility. Moreover, age has a direct impact on the success of any fertility-enhancing procedures including assisted reproductive techniques (ART). A detailed explanation of the possible mechanisms underlying decreased fertility in both sexes with aging is well demonstrated in Chapter 2.

As a peculiar feminine entity, polycystic ovarian syndrome (PCOS) is a good example of ovaries being different from testes. There are some PCOS-related clinical manifestations that had been detected, which showed a number of its molecular mechanisms and provided many new theoretical basis for clinical PCOS prevention and treatment as shown in Chapter 3. As an example of long-term complications, sometimes, PCOS is associated with metabolic disorders and insulin resistance that should be kept in mind by all gynecologists as shown in Chapter 4. Treatment of PCOS represents a continuous dilemma in modern gynecologic practice. New modalities of therapy whether medical or surgical are controversial according to the patient complaint and evidence-based medicine. The topic of PCOS proper management is discussed in detail in Chapter 5 from an infertility point of view.

Autophagyis is the natural, regulated, destructive mechanism of the cell that disassembles unnecessary or dysfunctional components. It is involved both in ovaries and testes. Experimental evidence has shown that autophagy is an active route in the process of cellular elimination. The human testes are exposed to various toxins and environmental factors including limited nutrient supplies, hypoxia, and some other stresses that would deleteriously affect the process of spermatogenesis. In this book, one can read the full chapter dedicated to autophagy in the human testes (Chapter 6).

Despite being a small-sized book, it has a clear message to increase orientation of all scientists interested in this field by similar and dissimilar issues in ovaries and testes, which will lead to a better understanding and management of both sexes particularly in the field of infertility.

Prof. Atef M. Darwish
Department of Obstetrics and Gynecology,
Women's Health University Hospital,
Faculty of Medicine,
Assiut University, Egypt

Chapter 1

Introductory Chapter: One-Stop Infertility Evaluation Unit

Atef Darwish and Essam-Eldn Mohamed

Additional information is available at the end of the chapter

http://dx.doi.org/10.5772/intechopen.69631

1. Introduction

It is a dream for most couples to have their own children as a part of their relationship. Infertility is a distressing and sensitive problem affecting 10–15% of couples worldwide [1]. It affects one couple in six [2]. WHO considered it a clinical disease of the reproductive system [3].

2. When is a couple infertile?

For healthy young couples without any treatment, the probability of getting pregnant per a reproductive cycle is about 20–25%. Their cumulative probabilities of conception are 60% within the first six months, 84% within the first year, and 92% within the second year of regular fertility-focused sexual activity [4]. There is no definite cutoff point to say when a couple is infertile. If the couple is young, this term is used if they fail to conceive after 1 year of having regular sexual intercourse without the use of birth control. Early evaluation can be started after 6 months if the female is older than 35 years. A known fertility medical problem or a social circumstance like previous prolonged infertility in a previous marriage of one of the partners is another indication for early evaluation.

3. Infertility is a real disease

Infertility, particularly if it is long term, is probably one of the most difficult times in a couple's life. Many physicians underestimate infertility problem, and this behavior is distressing to the infertile couple. The physician should be sympathetic with the patients and should be very keen and kind to solve this real problem. Infertility is usually associated with social stigma and can lead to divorces and separation, leading to a broken family life. Infertility generates disability (an impairment of function), and thus, access to health care falls under the Convention on the Rights of Persons with Disability. Infertility in women was ranked the fifth highest serious global disability [5].

4. Time limit to reach the diagnosis of infertility

In general, the cause of infertility can be found within one to two cycles in most cases (80–85% of cases) with the use of standard diagnostic measures like semen analysis (SA), tests for ovulation, and tubal patency. The rest is considered unexplained infertility (UI). UI does not mean there is no physical explanation for infertility, but it is just that medical tests have not identified any specific problems [6].

5. What are the additional complaints of the infertile couple?

In addition to failure to conceive, many infertile couples have extra complaints like failure to understand the main cause of their infertility, the stress of prolonged medical or hormonal treatment, fear of some operative procedures for the male or the female partner, stress of the surrounding community, and wasting time in the clinics and hospitals. Moreover, many doctors consider imperial lines of treatment relying on the natural percentage of pregnancy with time. Lengthy courses especially for the male make infertile couple drug-linked. Many cases develop Gastrointestinal tract (GIT) troubles on prolonged courses of drug therapy that may lead to discontinuation of therapy. Overoptimistic hope with strict following of instructions faints out due to nonoccurrence of pregnancy as the physician does not tell them the truth that the highest pregnancy rate/cycle is just 20%/cycle in most cases [7]. Lack of cooperation between gynecologists and andrologists makes one partner's treatment not synchronous with the other. In addition, gynecologic treatment for men is usually underestimated by the male partner.

6. Construction of an infertility unit: as a solution of most of the additional complaints

6.1. Rationale

A basic concept is to consider both partners as one unit. If the evaluation of both partners starts simultaneously, prompt diagnosis and short treatment pathway can be expected. Some gynecologists are poor at interpreting semen analysis reports or dealing with infertile men. The same applies for the andrologists regarding female investigations. Collaboration between gynecologists and andrologists would expand their knowledge about proper diagnostic as well as therapeutic approaches of the case.

6.2. Prerequisites

- **Team approach:** A well-trained team is a basic requirement for an efficient infertility unit. A team approach is the most successful and cut-short way to diagnose and promptly treat a case of infertility. A team approach is proposed to save a lot of time and money lost by trials and errors of lengthy medical treatment or unnecessary investigations. Evaluation requires a well-trained gynecologist, an andrologist, nurses, health providers, and a clinical pathologist. The investigators should not accuse one partner in front of the other partner that he or she is the main cause of infertility even if the examination or investigations show that he or she is the most probable cause of infertility. Accusing one partner will lead to many psychological upsets and will interfere with sexual activity. Nurses and health care providers should be trained on how to deal with the infertile couple who are usually injured by the failure of conception. Their job is very important as it saves the time of the clinicians. Stress on hygiene and coital recommendations should be highlighted. Even how and when to take injections, particularly hormones, is very important for better results. In short, the main goal of an infertility unit is to minimize time and effort to reach a diagnosis of infertility. All basic requirements to achieve this goal should be available at this unit including imaging modalities and laboratory equipment for hormonal assay.

- **Prepregnancy counseling:** Ideally, any couple willing to have children should be evaluated prior to allowing unprotected intercourse. Increased risk of congenital anomalies with increased maternal age should be highlighted. Some women may have some serious diseases that may contraindicate pregnancy. Some serious cardiac diseases like cardiomyopathy or heart failure are good examples. Some diseases require prepregnancy modification of the therapy prior to pregnancy. Diabetic women on oral hypoglycemic agents should be switched to insulin therapy prior to fertilization of the oocyte. Prepregnancy estimation of blood sugar and glycosylated hemoglobin is essential to have a good idea about control of diabetes and to estimate the possible risk of fetal anomalies. The same applies to the male partner. Men on antihepatitis drugs or chemotherapy or radiotherapy should be properly evaluated prior to allowance of pregnancy. If some chromosomal diseases are expected due to a past or family history of either partner, a thorough genetic and chromosomal workup is mandatory. In short, prepregnancy evaluation of both partners is an integral part of the infertility evaluation.

- **Check fertility awareness of the infertile couple:** This is a crucial job for the entire infertility team. Surprisingly, only 13% of women seeking fertility assistance could accurately identify the most fertile time in their menstrual cycle. It is possible that poor fertility knowledge could be a key factor in cases of infertility. Fertility education should be a fundamental part of preconception care and the primary care of couples when they first report difficulty conceiving. Intercourse on fertile days of the menstrual cycle may help in getting pregnant and avoid unnecessary Assisted Reproductive Techniques (ART) treatment [8]. Cervical mucus monitoring (CMM) can identify the fertile days with the highest pregnancy rate [9]. Timed intercourse may improve pregnancy rates compared to intercourse without ovulation prediction [10]. Basal body temperature chart poorly predicts ovulation. A single serum progesterone assessment in midluteal phase is as effective as repeated serum progesterone measures [11].

- **Optimizing natural fertility [12]:** Some physicians go directly into investigating couples, provided that they know natural fertility. Physicians should ask in detail about the basic knowledge of the couple on fertilization days. Frequent intercourse (daily or every other day) yields the highest pregnancy rates, but results achieved with less frequent intercourse (two to three times weekly) are nearly equivalent. The "fertile window" spans the 6-day interval ending on the day of ovulation and correlates with the volume and character of cervical mucus. Specific coital timing or position and resting supine after intercourse have no significant impact on fertility. For women having regular menstrual cycles, frequent intercourse should begin soon after cessation of help to maximize fecundability. The use of most commercially available vaginal lubricants should be discouraged for couples trying to conceive. Devices designed to determine or predict the time of ovulation may be useful for couples who have infrequent intercourse.

- **Have an idea about lifestyle and occupation of both couples:** Overexercise or sedentary life would affect fertility in both partners. Occupations with exposure to some chemicals like some pesticides, herbicides, metals (lead), and solvents have been linked to fertility problems in both men and women. Couples should be asked about continuous or daily traveling of either partner.

- **Direct inquiry about habits and addiction:** Smoking, recreational drugs and alcohol consumption are lifestyle factors that are suspected to have adverse effects on health and subsequently reproductive functions [13, 14]. It has been estimated that in each menstrual cycle, smokers have about two-third the chance of conceiving compared to nonsmokers. Smoking is also harmful to a developing baby if the mother smokes. For men, mostly due to defective oxygen supply, heavy smoking would lead to decreased sperm concentration, viability, motility, increased DNA fragmentation, and poor outcome of IVF/ICSI [15, 16]. Therefore, it is a good time for both partners to stop if they are smokers. There are many studies on the deleterious effects of recreational drugs, sports drugs (anabolic steroids), marijuana, opioids and tramadol on spermatogenesis in men, and folliculogenesis in women [17–20].

- **Focus on a fertility diet:** Women who become seriously underweight as a result of an eating disorder or severe anemia or vegans may have fertility problems. They should be promptly treated with suitable supplementation prior to pregnancy. Normal females should be advised to increase intake of some foods or drinks rich in multivitamins that are thought to support ovulation, hormonal balance, and oocyte quality. The male partner is also advised to improve his dietary habits. Good nutrition with diets rich in multivitamins would improve sperm motility and viability.

- **Searching for risk factors of infertility:** These factors can be obtained from history, examination, and investigations of both partners.

  History-taking: Ideally both partners should be seen together. Evaluation of both partners must begin with a detailed history-taking directed to complete all items related to infertility. It should be fertility-oriented history-taking, which means asking about any possible cause of infertility and any possible problem that may interfere with infertility treatment or subsequent pregnancy or delivery later on. Importantly to ask about past history of medical or surgical treatment of this current problem, this is actually a history of present illness. The most important part of taking an infertility history is to ask women and men of reproductive age if they are sexually active, if they are trying to get pregnant, and for how long they have been trying. Not all women will complain openly about their inability to get pregnant; instead, they may present with surrogate complaints such as lower abdominal pain or abnormal vaginal bleeding. A careful history can often help to find the causes of infertility. Gynecologists, as well as andrologists, should pay attention to the following clues:

Age: It is the most important independent factor of infertility due to changing ovulation patterns and reduced oocyte quality, and it is one of the most important prognostic factors for treatment outcome. For healthy, young couples, the chance that a woman will become pregnant is about 20% in any single menstrual cycle and starts to decline in a woman who is in her early 30s. It declines more rapidly after age 37 [7]. A woman has 12% of her ovarian reserve at age 30 and has only 3% at age 40. About 81% of the variation in ovarian reserve is due to age alone, making age the most important factor in female infertility. For women aged 35–39, the chance of conceiving is about half that of women aged 19–26 [21]. ACOG recommends ovarian reserve testing for women older than 35 years who have not conceived after 6 months of attempting to get pregnant and for women at higher risk of diminished ovarian reserve such as those with a history of cancer treated with genotoxic therapy, pelvic irradiation, or both; those with medical conditions who were treated with genotoxic therapies; or those who had ovarian surgery for endometriomas. It is important to recognize that a poor result from ovarian reserve testing does not signify an absolute inability to conceive and should not be the sole criterion considered to limit or deny access to infertility treatment [21]. An important point is that with aging there are higher percentages of chromosomal defects in the oocytes of older women, which may cause infertility, miscarriages, or Down syndrome in full-term babies. This defect can be attributed to poor working of the "glue" that keeps the chromosomes or poor function of the microtubules in the chromosomes. Instead of sending an even number to each oocyte in a controlled fashion, the microtubules go in all directions in old oocytes. So, it is not only a matter of decreased ovarian reserve but also poor-quality eggs. Likewise, it is thought that men over the age of 35 are half as likely to achieve a pregnancy when compared to men younger than 25. Levita et al. [22] examined 6022 semen samples according to WHO criteria and correlated findings to patients' age. They reported an inverse statistically significant correlation between semen volume, sperm quality, and patient age, in spite of prolonged sexual abstinence duration. Top sperm parameters were observed at the age of 30 to <35 years, while the most significant reduction in sperm parameters occurred after the age of 55.

Current drug therapy or medical illness: Many commonly used drugs, as well as cancer chemotherapeutic agents, are potentially toxic to the gonads [23]. There is a possible association between impaired semen qualities and the commonly used histamine H1-receptor antagonists, antiepileptic drugs, antibiotics, histamine H2-receptor antagonists, mast cell blockers, antidepressants, and brain stimulators [24]. Diabetes mellitus may affect male reproductive function at multiple levels as a result of its effects on the endocrine control of spermatogenesis or spermatogenesis itself or by impairing penile erection and ejaculation [25]. Renal failure impairs the endocrine system, especially in women, due to hyperprolactinemia, altering fertility, ovulation, libido, and growth in adolescents. Kidney transplant is less efficient for restoring the perfect function of the hypothalamic-pituitary-gonadal axis due in part to the immunosuppressant regimens prescribed [26].

- **Gynecological history:** Regular cycles are commonly ovulatory cycles. In a previous study, only 3.7% were proved an ovulatory despite regular eumenorrheic women [27]. Heavy regular menses may signify an intrauterine polyp or a submucous myoma. Irregular menses may signify ovarian dysfunction. Postcoital spotting or even bleeding may signify a local lesion in the cervix or vagina. Oligohypomenorrhea or even periods of amenorrhea responsive to progesterone challenge test signify ovarian factor. If associated with evidence of hyperandrogenism, the possibility of polycystic ovaries (PCOS) is raised. Failure to respond to progesterone and combined progesterone and estrogen tests may signify an end-organ failure like severe intrauterine adhesions. However, the possibility of undiagnosed pregnancy should always be kept in mind. Any form of dysmenorrhea should be recorded. Severe spasmodic dysmenorrhea may signify tight cervical stenosis or uterine malformation. Severe congestive dysmenorrhea may signify a uterine mass or severe pelvic inflammatory disease (PID).

- **Think endometriosis:** It is mentioned that you will not diagnose endometriosis unless you are endometriosis-oriented. Endometriosis is definitely associated with infertility; however, the mechanism of impaired fertility in the presence of minimal disease has not been clearly documented. Endometriosis is suspected whenever a special type of dysmenorrhea is present. It starts as congestive dysmenorrhea but continues during menses and subsides after few days when fluid is absorbed from the retained menstrual blood in the endometriotic lesion. Of course, dyspareunia especially the deep type raises the possibility of endometriosis.

- **Past medical and surgical history:** Start by asking about childhood development, sexual development during puberty, menarche, sexual history, or chronic illnesses. Moreover, please ask about prolonged medications especially immunosuppressant or chemotherapeutic drugs used; exposure to certain environmental agents (alcohol, radiation, steroids, chemotherapy, and toxic chemicals); and any previous fertility evaluations especially invasive procedures like HSG or laparoscopy. Attention should be directed to prior treatment for pelvic inflammatory diseases (PID) or STDs (for chlamydia, HPV, herpes, syphilis, or trichomonas), which may suggest tubal damage and pelvic adhesions. History of pulmonary tuberculosis or bilharziasis may raise the suspicion of genital tract damage, which may necessitate HSG or even laparoscopy [28]. Detailed history-taking of previous surgeries particularly pelvic surgery is mandatory as the nearer to the pelvis, the higher possibility of fertility affection by the surgery. Of great importance is to obtain details of the past history of appendectomy, ovarian cystectomy, myomectomy, or tubal surgery. Past history of uterine surgery can affect fertility by induction of intrauterine adhesions or cervical stenosis. The latter commonly occurs after cervical amputation or large loop excision of the transformation zone (LLETZ) in cases of abnormal cytology and colposcopy.

- **Obstetric history:** A detailed history of a previous delivery whether vaginally or by cesarean section is mandatory. Sometimes, intraoperative or postoperative complications may have a direct impact on future fertility. In such cases, investigations should focus on tubal, peritoneal, or uterine factors of infertility. Hysterosalpingography (HSG) or even combined laparoscopy and hysteroscopy should have a priority during investigating this couple. Ask about a course of previous pregnancies and deliveries with stress on any complication related to either of them. Sometimes, past history of serious pregnancy or delivery complication is considered as a contraindication for future pregnancy like an acute renal failure with repeated dialysis, placenta accrete on the scar, or repair of a ruptured uterus. In such cases, the health provider should convince the couple to avoid pregnancy for the sake of saving the woman's life. The same applies for women with recurrent miscarriages who may require investigation before they try to get pregnant again.

- **Male history:** Ask about pregnancies or deliveries by a previous wife or previous attempts to get pregnant via ART, previous sexually transmitted infections, mumps, or trauma to the scrotum.

- **Social history:** Infertility can have many negative social implications. The socioeconomic environment of the patient should be explored. A couple should have basic means to raise a child. In addition, resources for possible infertility investigations and treatment should be discussed.

- **Sexual history:** Many infertile subjects experienced trouble in various aspects of sexuality [29]. Couples may not volunteer such information unless specifically asked. For optimal fertility, couples should have intercourse every 2–3 days. Ask about frequency and timing of sexual relation, orgasm, lubrication in females, and desire and potency of the male. Ask about any difficulties with intercourse. Deep dyspareunia may suggest pelvic pathology. Impotence and vaginismus can also be causes of infertility [30]. In one of these situations, when they become imperative to have intercourse at specific times, some of them will be affected by poor erection. What was once an intimate moment can become very clinical and a job. Going into a sterile room with a cup, under the pressure of performance, can harm any male. Women undergoing infertility treatment experience significant changes in various aspects of sexual desire, arousal, orgasm, length of foreplay, and frequency of intercourse [31].

- **Stress factor of infertility:** A physician should be clever to observe couples with stress. Studies indicate that female ovulation and male sperm production may be affected by mental stress. If one partner is stressed, it will affect the quality and frequency of sexual intercourse, resulting in a lower chance of conception. It is thought that the more relaxed and spontaneous sexual life is, the more likely that conception will occur. Also, stress can affect libido and how often the couple has sex. Long cycles (32 days or longer) are usually associated with stress (emotional or physical). A systematic review [32] found that there is evidence that infertility has a negative effect on the psychological well-being and sexual relationships of couples, but the evidence is inconclusive for the effect on marital relationships and quality of life.

7. Examination of the infertile couple

Infertility evaluation should include a complete physical examination of the male and female partners, as well as an array of laboratory and imaging studies.

Consider **"testes and ovaries - functional and clinical differences and similarities"** during the examination of an infertile couple. Evaluate primary and secondary sexual organs in both partners. Ovarian and uterine measurements and volume by Transvaginal Ultrasonography (TVS) as well as testicular measurements and volume by clinical examination and by testicular ultrasonography would give a good idea about the primary sex organs. Small-sized gonads would suggest defective folliculogenesis or spermatogenesis as well as defective sex hormone production. Proper development of secondary sexual characters may reflect normal steroidogenesis. Poorly developed characters would suggest hypogonadism mostly due to an underlying genetic abnormality. In such cases, baseline hormonal profile is mandatory.

8. Fertility-oriented examination

The general examination is very essential from the fertility point of view. Focus on stature, body built, and look. Overweight or underweight female or male may affect fertility. Excessive facial or body hair, weight gain, or staring look may indicate hormonal imbalances that can impair ovulation. These findings are often found in PCOS and thyroid conditions. Oxidative stress, inflammation, and insulin resistance are common mediators of the effects of obesity on reproduction. Moreover, obesity is a prominent aggravating factor in the development of PCOS [33]. Meticulous breast examination in female and male partners for evidence of masses (gynecomastia in male) or galactorrhea should not be ignored as the latter may interfere with ovulation and implantation. Abdominal examination is done to document any scar of a previous operation that may interfere with fertility or interfere with infertility management like laparoscopy. Any abdominal masses should be thoroughly evaluated. Vaginal examination is essential to find out any local genital cause of infertility like chronic cervicitis, cervical masses, or polyps. Comment on the position of the cervix is helpful. If it is high and attracted upwards particularly after cesarean section, a possibility of uterine adhesions to the anterior abdominal wall is expected. In such cases, the investigator should go to laparoscopic evaluation faster than other investigations to perform ureterolysis and adhesiolysis of any associated adhesions. Male partner should be examined while standing with a comment on testicular size, evidence of hydrocele, varicocele, or epididymal cyst or nodules.

9. Fertility-oriented investigations

9.1. Hormonal assay

One of the clues to a successful one-stop infertility unit is to facilitate blood sampling for hormonal assay in the same place. Besides saving a lot of time and effort for the infertile couple, it avoids lab-to-lab discrepancies and allows frequent interactive discussion with the clinical pathologist to correlate clinical with laboratory findings. Basic hormonal profile should include FSH and LH. Serum prolactin (better fasting morning sample) and TSH are helpful particularly if the female has galactorrhea or irregular cycles. Free testosterone and specific suprarenal DHEA-sulfate are requested whenever excessive androgen or hirsutism is present. Day 21 serum progesterone is mandatory to confirm ovulation. AMH and FSH are good ovarian reserve tests if its compromise is suspected.

9.2. A quick guide to assessing semen analysis

In clinical settings, at least two semen samples should be obtained because of the significant intraindividual variation of semen parameters.

- **Old or recent SA report?** Previous SA reports should be evaluated in a chronologic manner. Take an overview on the homogeneity of reports. Exclude eccentric or poorly performed reports. Usually, they direct you toward a specific diagnosis by repetition of the same defective finding in all or most reports. A new SA is requested if you are confused with the previous reports, when they are old or heterogeneous, or if the male has a recent indication for SA. Repeatedly, normal SA excludes male factor.
- **Which WHO SA report?** Old WHO manual has many limitations. First, data were derived from imprecisely defined reference populations and obtained from laboratories with unknown comparability with respect to analytical methodologies. Second, there is a lack of available data on semen variables in recent fathers and they did not define true reference ranges or limits. In 2010, WHO changed guidelines for SA. A man with sperm

Finding	Main cause	Diagnostic steps	Management
Agglutination	Infection, antisperm antibodies	Culture, antisperm antibodies	Appropriate antibiotic
Acidic pH (<7.2–8)	Infection	Culture	Appropriate antibiotic
Oligospermia(<1.5 ml)	Poor collection, hypogonadism, or partial obstruction	Hormonal profile, ultrasonography	Repeat SA, causal
Oligozoospermia (<15 mil/ml)	Varicocele, smoking, leukospermia, or genetic abnormalities	Repeated semen analysis, serum testosterone level, and transrectal ultrasound (TRUS)	Treatment of the cause
Oligozoospermia, asthenozoospermia (progressive sperm motility<32%) **and/or teratozoospermia** (normal sperm morphology <4%)	Varicocele, smoking, leukospermia, or genetic abnormalities	Clinical examination, Doppler scrotal US	Treatment of the cause Antioxidants and/or anti estrogen
Pyospermia	Infection (s)	Prostatic culture and sensitivity	Appropriate antibiotic
Azoospermia	Spermatogenic arrest, genetic defect, or obstruction	Hormonal profile, scrotal US, TRUS, seminal fructose, α-glucosidase, genetic assessment	Treatment of the cause, epididymovasostomy or sperm retrieval and ICSI

count ≥15 million/ml, >4% normal morphology, and ≥40% progressive motility would be considered normal.

- **Quick guide for SA interpretation**

9.3. Imaging modalities

First-visit transabdominal as well as transvaginal ultrasonographic evaluation of the infertile female is very helpful to detect ovarian or uterine factors. Antral follicle count is a good ovarian reserve test. Folliculometry and comment on the endometrium are valuable, especially in ART programs. Scrotal US allows the differentiation of obstructive azoospermia (OA) (normal vessel distribution) from nonobstructive azoospermia (reduced or absent testicular vessels) [33]. Transrectal ultrasound (TRUS) enables high-resolution imaging of the prostate, seminal vesicles, and vas deferens and is the modality of choice in diagnosing congenital and acquired abnormalities implicated in the cause of obstructive azoospermia (OA). MRI is rarely needed in infertile women particularly in some endometriosis cases. Pituitary MRI may be requested if the pituitary adenoma is suspected. In men MRI is useful for both detection and characterization of prostatic cysts detected on a TRUS and evaluation of the vas deferens, seminal vesicles, and ejaculatory ducts.

9.4. Tubal patency testing

Think of tubal factor whenever your patient has a previous gynecologic or nongynecologic pelvic surgery or cesarean section, while other factors are normal or normal SA, ovulation, and hormonal profile without pregnancy. Consider the therapeutic effect of HSG during counseling. Most of the scientific societies including ASRM consider that the initial assessment of tubal patency is HSG [34]. Laparoscopy is restricted to cases with a history of pelvic surgery or history suggestive of pelvic endometriosis or patients with abnormal HSG. Saline infusion sonography (SIS) is a valuable easy office test without irradiation risks but less accurate than HSG.

9.5. Endoscopy

Combined laparoscopy and hysteroscopy are requested in selected cases [6].

9.6. Additional optional male investigation

Sperm DNA fragmentation (SDF) is valuable in cases with idiopathic infertility, excessive abnormal forms, or repeated abortions, while hypo-osmotic swelling test (HOST) has been proposed to test viability in severely immotile sperms or before ICSI.

9.7. Final step: treatment road map

At the end of one-stop evaluation of both partners, the team should decide the best treatment for each couple. A short meeting with the couple should explain the plan of management of infertility. Proper counseling regarding each option's advantages, disadvantages, and risks should be clarified.

9.8. Periodic team meetings

It is very important to assess the pattern and success of the provided service. Failures and successes should be discussed. Evidence-based discussion of every step is mandatory. Pitfalls in the diagnostic approaches should be corrected. Plan for further improvement should be clearly discussed. Local statistical analysis of the unit's results is very helpful.

10. Keynote points

- In the very fast modern world, construction of a one-stop infertility evaluation unit is recommended to cut-short lengthy infertility evaluation and treatment protocols and to widen the scope of both the gynecologist and andrologist.
- Gynecologists and andrologists should know how to disclose the male and female infertility factors, respectively, to counsel a future plan of investigations and management, and to provide actual prognostics figured for each individual case.

Author details

Atef Darwish[1]* and Essam-Eldn Mohamed[2]

*Address all correspondence to: atef_darwish@yahoo.com

1 Woman's Heath University Hospital, Assiut University, Assiut, Egypt

2 AlAzhar University, Assiut, Egypt

References

[1] Zargar AH, Wani AI, Masoodi SR, Laway BA, Salahuddin M. Epidemiologic and etiologic aspects of primary infertility in the Kashmir region of India. Fertility and Sterility. 1997;**68**:637-643

[2] Brugo-Olmedo S, Chillik C, Kopelman S. Definition and causes of infertility. Reproductive BioMedicine Online. 2001;**2**(1):41-53

[3] Zegers-Hochschild F, Adamson GD, de Mouzon J, Ishihara O, Mansour R, Nygren K, Sullivan E, van der Poel S on behalf of ICMART and WHO. The International Committee for Monitoring Assisted Reproductive Technology (ICMART) and the World Health Organization (WHO) revised glossary on ART terminology. Human Reproduction. 2009;**24**(11):2683-2687

[4] Kamel RM. Management of the infertile couple: An evidence-based protocol. Reproductive Biology and Endocrinology. 2010;**8**:21

[5] Abha K, Satendra S. Infertility: Why can't we classify this inability as disability? Australasian Medical Journal. 2012;**5**(6):334-339

[6] Darwish AM. Endoscopic explanation of unexplained infertility. In: Darwish A, editor. Contemporary Gynecologic Practice. Chapter 1. InTech Pub, Croatia; 2015

[7] ACOG FAQ. Evaluating Infertility. 2012

[8] Hampton KD, Mazza D, Newton JM. Fertility-awareness knowledge, attitudes, and practices of women seeking fertility assistance. Journal of Advanced Nursing. 2013;**69**(t5):1076-1084

[9] Thijssen A, Meier A, Panis K, Ombelet W. Fertility awareness-based methods and subfertility: A systematic review. Facts, Views and Vision in ObGyn. 2014;**6**(3):113-123

[10] Manders M, McLindon L, Schulze B, Beckmann MM, Kremer JA, Farquhar C. Timed intercourse for couples trying to conceive. The Cochrane Database of Systematic Reviews. 2015;(3):CD011345

[11] Guermandi E, Vegetti W, Bianchi M, Uglietti A, Ragni G, Grosignani P. Reliability of ovulation tests in infertile women. Obstetrics and Gynecology. 2001;**97**(1):92-96

[12] Practice Committee of the American Society for Reproductive Medicine in collaboration with the Society for Reproductive Endocrinology and Infertility. Optimizing natural fertility. Fertility and Sterility 2008;**90**(3):S1-S8

[13] Vine MF. Smoking and male reproduction: A review. International Journal of Andrology. 1996;**19**:323-337

[14] Kovac JR, Khanna A, Lipshultz LI. The effects of cigarette smoking on male fertility. The Postgraduate Medical. 2015;**127**(3):338-341

[15] Martini AC, Molina RI, Estofán D, Senestrari D, Fiol de Cuneo M, Ruiz RD. Effects of alcohol and cigarette consumption on human seminal quality. Fertility and Sterility. 2004;**82**:374-377

[16] Ricci G, Cacciola G, Altucci L, Meccariello R, Pierantoni R, Fasano S, Cobellis G. Endocannabinoid control of sperm motility: The role of the epididymis. General and Comparative Endocrinology. 2007;**153**:320-322

[17] Adam ML, Sewing B, Forman JB, Mever ER, Cicero TJ. Opioid induced suppression of testicular function in rats. The Journal of Pharmacology and Experimental Therapeutics. 1993;**266**:323-328

[18] Aloisi AM, Aurilio C, Bachioccco V, Biasi G, Fiorenzani P, Pace MC, Paci V, Pari G, Passavanti G, Ravaioli L, Sindaco G, Vellucci R, Ceccarelli I. Endocrine consequences of opioid therapy. Psychoneuroendocrinology. 2009;**34**(Suppl 1):S162-S168

[19] Ahmed MA, Kurkar A. Effects of opioid (tramadol) treatment on testicular functions in adult male rats: The role of nitric oxide and oxidative stress. Clinical and Experimental Pharmacology and Physiology. 2014;**41**(4):317-323

[20] Wallace WH, Kelsey TW. Human ovarian reserve from conception to the menopause. PLoS One. 2010;**5**(1):e8772

[21] ACOG. Committee opinion no. 618: Ovarian reserve testing. Obstetrics and Gynecology. 2015;**125**:268-273

[22] Levita E, Lunenfeld E, Weisz N, Friger M, Potashnik G. Relationship between age and semen parameters in men with normal sperm concentration: Analysis of 6022 semen samples. Andrologia. 2007;**39**(2):45-50

[23] Schlegel PN, Chang TS, Marshall FF. Antibiotics: Potential hazards to male fertility. Fertility and Sterility. 1991;**55**:235-242

[24] Hayashi T, Miyata A, Yamada T. The impact of commonly prescribed drugs on male fertility. Human Fertility (Cambridge). 2008;**11**(3):191-196

[25] Sexton WJ, Jarow JP. Effect of diabetes mellitus upon male reproductive function. Urology. 1997;**49**(4):508-513

[26] Atallah D, Salameh C, El Kassis N, Safi J, Lutfallah F, Bejjani L, Ghaname W, Moukarzel M. Infertility and kidney transplantation. Le Journal Médical Libanais. 2015;**63**(3):138-143

[27] Malcolm CE, Cumming DC. Does anovulation exist in eumenorrheic women? Obstetrics and Gynecology. 2003;**102**(2):317-318

[28] Darwish A. Laparoscopic evidence of upper genital schistosomiasis. Journal of Obstetrics and Gynaecology. 1999;**19**(2):122-124

[29] Tao P, Coates R, Maycock B. The impact of infertility on sexuality: A literature review. Australasian Medical Journal. 2011;**4**(11):620-627

[30] Volgsten H, Skoog A, Ekselius SL, Lundkvist O, Poromaa IS. Prevalence of psychiatric disorders in infertile women and men undergoing *in vitro* fertilization treatment. Human Reproduction. 2008;**23**(9):2056-2063

[31] Luk BH, Loke AY. The impact of infertility on the psychological well-being, marital relationships, sexual relationships, and quality of life of couples: A systematic review. Journal of Sex and Marital Therapy. 2015;**41**:610-625

[32] Georgopoulos NA, Saltamavros AD, Vervita V, Karkoulias K, Adonakis G, Decavalas G, Kourounis G, Markou KB, Kyriazopoulou V. Basal metabolic rate is decreased in women with polycystic ovary syndrome and biochemical hyperandrogenemia and is associated with insulin resistance. Fertility and Sterility. 2009;**92**:250-255

[33] Schurich M, Aigner F, Frauscher F, Pallwein L. The role of ultrasound in assessment of male fertility. The European Journal of Obstetrics and Gynecology and Reproductive Biology. 2009;**144**(Suppl 1):S192-S198

[34] The Practice Committee of the American Society for Reproductive Medicine. Optimal evaluation of the infertile female. Fertility and Sterility. 2006;**86**(5 Suppl):S264-S267

Chapter 2

The Impact of Aging on Fertility: Similarities and Differences between Ovaries and Testes

Alice Ioana Albu and Dragos Albu

Additional information is available at the end of the chapter

http://dx.doi.org/10.5772/intechopen.68905

Abstract

The increasing age seems to have a negative impact on reproductive functions not only in women but also in men. Therefore, our aim was to review the data available in the literature regarding the impact of advancing age on fertility and the mechanisms underlying this association in both genders. The available data suggest that the effects of age on ovarian function cause a decrease in fertility starting 13 years before menopause. Statistics show that 10% of women will have a decreased fertility starting with the age of 30. The impact of age on ovary is due to both decreased number and quality of the oocytes, resulting in a high rate of chromosomal aneuploidy in the embryo and mitochondria dysfunction. Assisted reproductive technologies aiming to identify competent embryo were created but for the moment the results are unsatisfactory. On the other hand, in men, the semen quality and testicular function were found to gradually decrease with age and most of the studies also describe a negative impact on fertility. The mechanisms underlying decreased fertility are mainly genetic and epigenetics changes. However, if the effects of age on male fertility in men can be overcome by assisted reproductive technologies is not clear yet as the results of the studies are inconsistent.

Keywords: aging, male fertility, female fertility

1. Introduction

The increasing age has a negative effect on reproductive function not only in women but also in men. This aspect seems to gain importance since in the last decades; there is a trend to an increased age in both genders at the first pregnancy. While the decreasing reproductive potential of women with age is well known, the modification of the reproductive function in men with increasing age is not entirely understood. The lack of a clear definition of an advanced reproductive paternal age and the mechanisms involved interfere with adequate counselling of the couple regarding future fertility. Therefore, our aim was to review the data available in the literature regarding the impact of advancing age on fertility and the mechanisms underlying this association in both genders.

1.1. Methods

We performed a review of the available data regarding the impact of advanced age on fertility in both men and women. We searched in PubMed and Google Scholar using the following key words: maternal age, paternal age, ovarian aging, fertility, infertility, chromosome aberrations, reproduction, pregnancy, pregnancy complications, assisted reproduction, ovary, and testes. Only articles written in English and French were selected.

2. Aging and fertility in men

2.1. Trend of increasing paternal age

A study published in 2006 showed an increase in paternal age over 2 decades among British couples from 29.2 years in 1980 to 32.1 years in 2002 [1, 2]. Moreover, the proportion of fathers aged 35–54 years increased from 25 in 1993 to 40% over 10 years [1]. These data probably parallel a worldwide change in reproductive dynamic, reflecting societal changes: couples start their families later waiting for a more favorable socio-economic environment and taking into account the change in women's role in society and increased access to reproductive technologies. However, the exact impact on fertility and health of the offspring because of this increase in paternal age is not completely understood, although some studies suggest detrimental effects.

Although the effect of delaying time of conception in women is extensively studied and strategies to counteract the negative consequences on the fetus are available, the potential effect of increasing age on male fertility has just started to be evaluated. While early studies failed to find an association between higher paternal age and infertility [3, 4], recent studies suggest a detrimental effect of increasing age on a chance to conceive. In one study published in 2000, couples with pregnancies of at least 24 weeks of gestation had a decreased chance of pregnancy within 12 months in comparison with men younger than 25 years (or 0.62 for men who are 30–34 years old, 0.5 for men who are 35–39 years old, and 0.51 for men ≥40 years old) [5]. Moreover, the increased paternal age seems to interact with the maternal age as suggested by the study of de La Rochbrochard and Thonneau which showed that men older than 40 years had an increased risk of infertility in couples with women older than 35 years [6]. Similarly, the study of Hassan and Killick confirmed that men older than 45 years associate with a decreased chance to achieve pregnancy within 1 year, in comparison to men younger than 25 years. [7].

The decline in male fertility with advancing age could be explained by several mechanisms. First of all, sexual dysfunction is one of the possible contributors as the frequency of the sexual intercourse significantly decreases with age and can significantly impact the fertility [8, 9]. Furthermore, semen parameters and testosterone levels can be altered with advancing age and an increased number of genetic abnormalities could appear.

The decline in testosterone levels as men age has been consistently reported in cross-sectional [10, 11] and longitudinal studies [12–17]. However, the clinical significance of this decline and the utility of testosterone administration are not completely clarified. Whether this process is part of the physiological aging or is influenced by other factors (potentially correctable) is also a subject of research. A longitudinal study published in 2013 comprising 2736 community-dwelling men aged 40–79 years [18] demonstrated that the age-related changes in testosterone levels could be influenced by lifestyle modifications: weight loss was associated with a proportional increase and weight gain with a proportional decrease in testosterone, free testosterone, and sex hormone-binding globulin (SHBG). Moreover, smoking cessation was related to a greater decline in testosterone in comparison to smokers. The number of comorbid conditions or physical activities did not seem to have an influence on hypothalamic-pituitary-testicular (HPT) axis function [18]. However, this study, in agreement with the previous studies, confirmed the modest decline of testosterone and free testosterone with age, while SHBG and luteinizing hormone (LH) increased, although the mean values of hormones remain within normal ranges.

Although the testosterone level decreases with age, only a small proportion of aging men present with testosterone levels below the normal range are being diagnosed with late onset hypogonadism. Among subjects included in the European Male Aging Study (EMAS), the prevalence of late onset hypogonadism was of 2.1 among men over 40 years old and 5.1% among men over 70 years old [19].

This decrease in testosterone levels seems to be the consequence of a decline in testicular and hypothalamic function with age. Histopathological postmortem studies support this hypothesis showing a reduced number of Leydig cells (~44% lower in men aged 50–76 than in men aged 20–48) [20]. It was also demonstrated that the Leydig cells responsiveness to LH administration is decreased in older men [21]. An exaggerated response of gonadotropin-releasing hormone (GnRH) to the negative feedback of testosterone and estrogen was also suggested to be involved in hypogonadism of older men [22].

However, the decrease in testosterone levels in aging men is not universally found, being probably influenced by numerous factors. A study published in 2010 demonstrated an association between polymorphisms in genes related to the pituitary-testicular endocrine function and circulating LH, testosterone, and estradiol levels [23].

Whether this decrease in testicular function has an impact on spermatogenesis is an interesting aspect which needs further clarification, taking into account the close correlation between gonadal steroids and spermatogenic functions in men.

The reports about changes of semen parameters with increasing age started in 1970 and many studies were published until today. Most of these studies found a decrease of semen volume, percentage of motile spermatozoa, and of normal morphology [24–26]. In turn, sperm concentration was reported to be unchanged [27], decreased [26], and even increased with advancing age [28] in healthy men. On the other hand, studies on infertile men demonstrated an unaltered [29] or an increase in sperm concentration [28]. However, most of these studies included a limited number of older subjects, making difficult to analyze the impact of aging on semen parameters. The study by Brahem et al. [30] demonstrated an effect of age of decreasing semen volume and vitality only in infertile patients in comparison with men with proven fertility. In contrast, the sperm concentration significantly increased with age [30]. The alteration of sperm parameters with age could be due to age-related histological changes observed in the testis. For instance, a study of the testes of 26 postmortem male subjects aged 16–80 years found a significant decline in the number of Sertoli cells with age [31]. Another histological study showed that subjects over 50 years old have a decreased number of Sertoli cells and failure of spermatogenic cell development evident from the spermatid level. However, an increased apoptosis index and a decreased proliferation index were observed only in men over 70 years [32].

The age-related decline in semen parameters could be also determined by the deterioration of the function of the seminal vesicle (contributing to ejaculate volume), prostate, and epididymis [33].

2.2. The genetic modifications during aging

2.2.1. DNA fragmentation

The results of a meta-analysis, including 26 studies and 10,220 patients, showed an increased DNA fragmentation paralleling advancing age [34]. The study by Moskovtsev et al. [35] evaluated infertile men, showing that the DNA fragmentation index increased gradually from 15.2 in men <30 years to 19.4, 20.1, 26.4, and 32.0% in men in the age groups 30–35, 35–40, 40–45, and over 45 years [35]. The association between DNA fragmentation and increasing age was also found in men with normozoospermia and oligoasthenoteratozoospermia [36].

Sperm DNA fragmentation seems to be an important determinant of fertility since it was reported to be associated with a reduced chance to conceive, a higher time of conception [37–39], and poorer outcomes in intrauterine insemination and IVF (in vitro fertilisation)/ ICSI (intracytoplasmic sperm injection) [40–44]. Moreover, it is possible that altered sperm DNA integrity has an impact on early embryonic development according to studies reporting a reduction of embryo morphokinetic parameters [45, 46], a reduced implantation rate, [47] and a poor embryo's post-implantation development resulting in pregnancy loss [48]. The study of Sivanarayana et al. [49] showed that sperms with abnormal forms (elongated, thin, round, pyri, amorphous, micro-, and macro-forms) and abnormal motility parameters were significantly associated with a higher DNA fragmentation index [49]. Therefore, the selection of morphologically normal spermatozoa for ICSI procedure could provide a possible explanation for the divergent results of studies evaluating the association of DNA fragmentation and ICSI outcome.

2.2.2. Aneuploidies

Chromosomal aberrations are frequently found in human gametes (21% of oocytes and 9% of spermatozoa) [50], with a predominance of aneuploidies in oocytes, whereas structural chromosomal abnormalities predominate in spermatozoa. Chromosomes 21, 22, and 16 are usually overrepresented in aneuploid gametes. In turn, sex chromosomes are particularly prone to non-disjunction in human sperm. Whereas the frequency of aneuploidy seems to be increased in infertile male sperm [33], the advanced paternal age is not convincingly associated with the presence of aneuploid sperms [50, 51]. Except an increased risk for trisomy 21, there are contradictory evidences for trisomy 18, 13, 47 XXY, and 45X [52] associated with paternal age. Bosch et al. [53] also reported a positive linear association of age with the structural and numerical abnormalities of chromosome 9 in sperm of the healthy donors, but these findings are limited by the reduced number of subjects (n = 18) [53]. A study published in 2011 reviewed the data on the association between paternal age and the presence of aneuploidy in sperms and concluded that in spite of decades of research and ''innumerable microscope hours", the literature is inconclusive [54]. The authors suggested that a low efficacy of FISH (fluorescence in situ hybridization) in detecting aneuploidies can be involved in the results of the studies and proposed that the array-based approaches will be a better method in addressing the question of a paternal age effect [54]. However, other methodological problems of the previous papers can be also involved as the number of patients was quite small in most of the studies and the age range was not always wide enough to be able to detect an association. A study published in 2005, evaluating testicular samples of subjects aged 29–102 years, reported that spermatogenesis is not invariably affected by age and the frequency of aneuploidies is increased only in older individuals with arrested spermatogenesis, suggesting an interaction between these two conditions [55]. An experimental study on mice also observed an association of increased age not only with sex chromosomal disomy and a high rate of germ cell apoptosis but also a high inter-individual variability in germ cell apoptosis. The authors concluded that the compromised apoptosis could contribute to high aneuploidies rate observed in older mice [56].

The study by De Souza et al. [57] showed that older fathers have an increased risk of having children with Klinefelter syndrome and XYY syndrome [57], in accordance with the described paternal origin of these sex chromosomes. Although slightly, the risk of Patau and Edwards syndromes was also increased. Arnedo et al. reported that the paternal age was associated with a higher frequency of sperm XY disomy only in fathers with paternally inherited Klinefelter syndrome offspring [58].

Trisomy 21 is the most common trisomy in newborns, and it is clearly related to increased maternal age. Surprisingly, the risk for Down syndrome seems to be negatively related to paternal age according to a study reporting a double risk for Down syndrome in all maternal age groups for younger fathers [59]. On the other hand, another study showed that paternal age is positively associated with a high risk for Down syndrome only when mothers are older than 35 [60]. However, the overall paternal contribution to Down syndrome appearance seems to be low as only in 5–10% of cases, excess 21 chromosome is of paternal origin [61].

Older studies reported no relationship between paternal age and autosomal trisomies [62, 63] or even a decreased risk of trisomy 13 for men older than 39 years [64] in comparison to a younger age group.

A recently published study evaluating the influence of the paternal age on the aneuploidies rates in embryos obtained from donated oocytes found that men older than 50 years had higher aneuploidy rates in embryos compared to the groups of men younger than 39 years and between 40–49 years old [65].

2.3. Abnormalities of the chromosomal structure

Due to the continuous process of spermatogenesis during the lifetime of a man, the spermatogonia are prone to an increased risk of mutations through a high number of cell divisions. This process could be aggravated with increasing age due to the toxic effect of oxidative stress and decreased DNA repair capacity [66, 67]. Moreover, increased paternal age is considered one of the major sources of mutations in humans [66].

2.4. Telomere length

Telomeres are regions of repetitive nucleotide sequences found at the end of the chromosomes, which have the function to protect the end of the chromosome from deterioration or from fusion with other chromosomes. Telomere length shortens with age and is associated with aging-related disorders. Telomere length decreases with every replication and, when a critical length is reached, cell division stops and cellular death appears. Although telomere shortening is considered to be related to advanced age and senescence [68], several studies reported a longer leucocytes telomere length in offspring of older fathers [69]. These findings are consistent with the longer telomere length reported in a subset of the sperm of older men. Probably this aspect is due to the selection of a particular germline stem cell subtype during the aging process with prolonged survival [69] but at the same time with affected mechanisms of healthy sperm selection [36].

The mechanisms connecting paternal age and telomere length of the offspring are not clearly elucidated. Although genome-wide association studies identified a number of genes linked to telomere length in general population, it is unlikely that increased number of mutations appearing with age in the paternal germline is the explanation for the observed association due to the rarity of these mutations [70].

One possible explanation is the age-dependent selection pressure in the male germline cells, older individuals having sperms with longer telomeres due to the selection process. This hypothesis is sustained by studies reporting a predominance of the sperm with longer telomers in older men [69].

Another hypothesis is offered by the different telomerase activities in somatic and germ-line cells. As such, telomerase is repressed in most somatic cells, whereas its activity is sustained in male germ-line stem cells [71]. Although the role of telomerase is to maintain the length of telomeres, after every replication of male germinal cells, a small increase with few base pairs seems to appear [72]. Due to the high number of replications of the germinal male cells over the life span, these small elongations accumulate, resulting in a significant increase of the telomere length in sperms of older men [70].

While most of the studies evaluated the relationship between paternal age and leucocytes telomere length, the positive correlation between paternal age and offspring sperm telomere length was for the first time reported in 2013 by a study evaluating a small sample (81 subjects) of young men (18–19 years old) [73]. However, in this study, the maternal age was also positively correlated to sperm telomere length, and the contribution of each parents' age was difficult to established due to the high correlation between parents age. They also found that sperm telomere length is related to sperm count, being lower in oligozoospermic than in normozoospermic men. These results confirmed the findings of Thilagavathi et al. [74] which reported shorter sperm telomere length in men with idiopathic infertility in comparison with controls [74]. Therefore, the number of studies linking infertility and low sperm count to shorter sperm telomere length is limited, and the question whether shorter sperm telomere length is the cause of infertility (through increased apoptosis of germ cells, impaired spermatogenesis, and reduced sperm count) or a marker of damaged spermatogenesis is yet to be answered by future studies.

Moreover, a study published in 2015 [75] reported a marked increase in sperm telomere length heterogeneity as men age and a longer length in samples with normal parameters in comparison with samples with abnormal parameters. These findings could have implications for infertile couples treated with assisted reproduction techniques due to a high probability of shorter telomere length in the offspring, taking into account the reported association between shorter telomere and depression, autism, neoplasia, and general poor health.

The exact implication of the paternal age at conception on the offspring health is not completely understood. Although it was generally considered to have a negative impact through the association with rare conditions like achondroplasia, Marfan syndrome, autism, and schizophrenia, it is also possible to be associated with a reduced risk of atherosclerosis and increased survival as longer telomere length confer this advantage [70].

Although telomere length is a complex genetic trait [76], several studies reported a possible impact of many other factors on telomere length like obesity, sleep disorders, smoking, and socio-economic factors, making the study the relationship between parental age and telomere length even more complicated.

2.5. Epigenetics

Data on the epigenetic changes related to paternal age are limited and refer mainly to modifications of methylation patterns observed in rats [77] and are considered to be involved in the appearance of Huntington disease, Alzheimer's disease, autism, or schizophrenia in humans [33].

3. Aging and fertility in women

Ovarian aging is a complex phenomenon that involves not only the reproductive function of the woman but also her global health status. Aging is characterized by a reduced number of oocytes and decreased fertility. Ovarian failure at menopause is associated with cardiovascular diseases, cognitive dysfunction, depression, and osteoporosis. The heat intolerance and hot flushes affect the quality of women life. Menopause is the final event in ovarian aging, with a mean age of occurrence of 51 years for the Caucasian population, with a range of individual variations due to genetic and environmental factors. Menopause is preceded by pre-menopause, a period that can last up to 10 years, characterized by a marked decline in fertility. The human follicles dynamic undergoes tremendous changes during this period, represented by a high rate of follicular atresia and a low rate of follicular growth, followed by exhaustion of follicular reserve, and, finally, occurrence of menopause.

The status of the women nowadays is changing, moving from high mortality and high fecundity to low mortality and low fecundity. There are remarkable changes in the dynamic of the world population and in the age distribution. It is estimated that in 2025, the number of women over 60 years old will equal the number of women 15–24 years, reversing the actual status [78]. Moreover, there is a continuous increase in the number of employed women which, in association with the increase in educational demands of women, will contribute to the postponed age of maternity. Therefore, current trends of the society determine an increased number of women to try to conceive at an older age. This decision generates a serious health problem due to the decreased fertility and a high rate of pregnancy complications associated with advanced age. The statistics show that the fertility is decreased by 31% in women, 35–39 years old, in comparison with women who are 20–24 years, and the same decrease in fertility is mirrored by the success in assisted reproductive techniques [79].

The epidemiological studies reflect these societal changes, reporting an increase in the age of women at first birth from 22.7 in 1980 to 28.2 years in 2003 [80]. This change in the maternal age at first birth is relevant, taking into account that women over 30 years old who had not yet conceived had lower chances to obtain pregnancy than women who previously conceived at younger ages [80].

Ovarian aging implies qualitative and quantitative alteration of ovarian reserve and a consecutive decline in fertility. In women, the ovarian pool, which is formed during intrauterine life, is gradually depleted and the number of oocyte aneuploidies are gradually increasing with age. Therefore, the number of miscarriages and implantation failure are rising with age. The ovarian pool gradually declines, but there are some crucial steps at 34, 37, and 40 years when the decline accelerates. This ovarian pool is not subsequently renewed [81].

The age-related decline in follicle number is bi-exponential but doubles beyond a critical point at the age of 37.5, when the number of follicles became less than 25,000 [82, 83]. From this point till menopause, the time interval is around 13 years, this time period being characterized by a decline in fertility (a subfertility status). If we consider women who enter menopause at 45 years, the cut-off value of less than 25,000 follicles will be reached at the age of 32. From a statistical point of view, 10% of women will enter menopause at 45 years, so there is 10% of women in the population who could potentially present subfertility since 32 years[84].

During intrauterine life, the ovary comprises 6 millions of oocytes surrounded by granulosa somatic cells, but because of atresia, only 1 million of primordial follicles remain at birth. At menarche, only 3,00,000 oocytes are left. During the female lifespan, approximately 400–500 follicles will ovulate [85].

Assisted reproduction technology had poor results in cases of ovarian aging, raising the economical, medical, and social cost of the procedures. On the other hand, oocyte donation programs have difficulties in finding donors. Social freezing of the oocytes creates various financial and storage problems and involves ethical issues and unequal access to medical care.

Ovarian aging is a complex process that implies genetic modifications and metabolic changes, causing a decreased competence of the oocytes to become a viable embryo that could implant and ovulate. Aging is associated with chromosomal aberrations of the oocytes, an increase in ovarian DNA fragmentation, a shortening of the ovarian telomere length, a decreased mitochondrial function, dysfunction of the granulosa cells, and a decreased testosterone production by the ovary. The use of Fourier transform infrared spectroscopy (FTIR) showed meaningful macromolecular and biochemical changes in human ovaries. The decline in ovarian quality with age was associated with important modifications on composition and distribution of all principal biomolecules: proteins, lipids, carbohydrates, and nucleic acids.

During the developmental stages of folliculogenesis, the oocyte growth is accompanied by the proliferation and differentiation of the granulosa cells. At the antral stage, the granulosa cells differentiate in two very different phenotypically populations: the cumulus granulosa cells (CGCs) and the mural granulosa cells. The CGCs are involved in oocyte growth and maturation and the mural granulosa cells are responsible for steroidogenesis [86, 87]. There are gap junctions between the CGCs and the oocyte. The accumulation of damages in granulosa cells during the long quiescent phase before entering the growing phase, or the alteration of cross-talk between granulosa cells and oocyte, contributes to the impact of aging on oocyte [87].

Both the oocytes and primordial follicles could stay in the ovary till the fifth decade and then start to grow and form mature oocytes. 60% of women over 40 remain infertile, comparable with 6% at the age group 20–24 [88]. The chance of pregnancy in a cycle is 30% for women between 27–29 years and 15% for women between 37–39 years. Natural delivery can occur after 45 years also but represents only 0.2% of total deliveries. However, most of the women that conceive at this age are multiparous [89]. It seems that the highest quality oocytes are used in the early reproductive years, leaving the less-competent oocytes for the fifth decade [90]. The chromosomal aberrations in the older ovaries are responsible for the increased number of embryo aneuploidies and miscarriages.

Kalmbach et al. [91] proposed the telomere shortening in the female germline as a central mechanism of reproductive aging in women [91]. The arguments for their theory are the studies on mice that demonstrated an association of telomere shortening with increases embryo fragmentation, cell cycle arrest, apoptosis, and chromosome abnormalities [92, 93]. In humans, it was reported that shorter telomeres in the oocytes of women undergoing in vitro fertilization were linked to the presence of fragmented, aneuploid embryos that fail to implant [94].

Mitochondria represent the powerhouse of the cells, producing the energy necessary for cellular functions. The ATP required for cellular energetic needs is produced by mitochondrial oxidative phosphorylation (OXPHOS). A toxic product of OXPHOS is endogenous reactive oxygen species (ROS). Natural defense mechanisms protect the cells against the damages produced by ROS, but if these mechanisms are decreased, the cells could be damaged. In the ovary, ROS may be involved in the regulation of follicular development or apoptosis through the modulation of ROS scavenging systems [95].

The theory of the free radicals' role in ovarian aging, which is 50 years old, says that these free radicals progressively accumulate with age and determine damages of the ovarian compartments and the decrease in ovarian function [96]. The evidences for this old theory are provided by studies showing a significant increase in oxidatively damaged lipids, proteins, and DNA [97] and a decrease in antioxidant defense in aging ovary [98, 99].

The increase of oxidative stress with ovarian aging could contribute to follicular atresia and a poor quality of oocytes as well [98]. Moreover, oxidative stress damages the telomeres and accelerates their shortening.

Mitochondria have their own genome in the form of mtDNA. This DNA is unstable in aging ovary. The maternal transmission of mtDNA is well established, and paternal transmission of mtDNA is being seen only in some pathological cases. Oocytes have a well-defined role in eliminating paternal mtDNA, but this ability has decreased in poor quality oocytes. The close relationship observed between mitochondrial dysfunctions and poor reproductive performance, which could be solved by injection of healthy mitochondria from another woman, led to the concept that the age of the ovary is related to the age of the mitochondrial function. Other signs of ovarian aging are point mutations or deletions of mitochondrial DNA.

Another theory is referring to the carbonyl stress in the aging follicle. Reactive carbonyl species (RCS) are reactive endogenous metabolites derived from metabolic processes. Unlike ROS, the damages produced by the RCS to the cells are more severe due to the increased stability of these products and their ability to attach to targets far from the site of their formation [100]. RCS determine post-translational modifications which finally form advanced glycation end-products (AGEs). Between AGEs and oxidative stress, there is a complex interplay with oxidative stress contributing to AGEs production [101].

These products accumulate in the ovary and promote the wide spatiotemporal spread of oxidative stress. These modifications affect the ovarian microenvironment during folliculogenesis, influencing the developmental capacity of the oocytes. It was also suggested that AGEs produce perturbation in perifollicular vascularization by a complex relationship with vascular endothelial growth factor (VEGF) [102, 103]. Therefore, the maturation, chromosomal constitution of the oocytes, and granulosa cell metabolism are modified. The granulosa cells are affected by oxidative stress including the glycosylation end products, resulting in a decrease in proliferation and an increase in apoptosis of the cells. Proteins modified by AGEs interact with specific receptors (RAGE) and through them determine the activation of the cell's response. The soluble RAGE could be measured in the follicular fluid and in the serum, and this is the method for quantifying the role of AGEs in ovarian aging and ovarian dysfunction. The study of Sato et al. [104] demonstrated that toxic AGE level in follicular fluid and in serum is negatively correlated with follicular growth, fertilization, and embryonic development [104].

One of the first endocrinological markers of ovarian aging is the early rise in day 3 follicle-stimulating hormone (FSH), together with the early elevation in estradiol levels and a more rapid growth of the follicles. First, there is a shortening of the follicular phase of the ovary and, later in the aging process, it is affected by the length of luteal phase and the value of serum luteal progesterone. Higher day 3 FSH level generally correlates with lower ovarian reserve and lower chances for pregnancy, the exception being FSH receptor variant. The cut-off value for subfertile population is generally considered a serum FSH of 12.3 UI/l. Other two markers of ovarian aging are antimullerian hormone (AMH) and antral follicle counts (AFC). AFC could be visualized by transvaginal ultrasonography, but the way AFC is performed differs between the centers. There are centers measuring follicles between 2–10 mm and others measuring follicles between 2–6 mm. It seems that smaller follicles, less than 6 mm, correlate better with ovarian reserve. In ART (assisted reproductive technology) literature, a lower AFC is associated with poor response to ovarian stimulation, although variable cut-offs were used, usually less than six. It was suggested that AFC is a better marker of ovarian reserve than AMH due to the factors potentially influencing circulating level of AMH (for instance, obesity). For AMH, the cut-off value for subfertility is considered 1 ug/l (Singer). It was also suggested that the response to ovarian stimulation during ART is a predictor of menopause based on the observation that women with a poor response experience early menopause and show menstrual cycle characteristics seen in ovarian aging. For the evaluation of the fertility potential of the women, it is important not only the age but also the number of years that elapse till menopause. At this moment, there is no gold standard for evaluating functional ovarian age. It seems that FSH-stimulated serum inhibin B level correlates best with ovarian age [105]. This stimulated serum inhibin B level reflects the pool of immature follicles, those not visible by ultrasound and not capable of estradiol production. With age the pool of immature follicles decreases accompanied by a decrease of serum level of inhibin B.

Very interestingly, in women with polycystic ovary syndrome (PCOS) with aging, the regular cycles are more regular, serum androgen levels decrease, and insulin resistance is ameliorated. In this case, the diminished pool of growing antral follicles determines a decrease in the AMH level. Women with PCOS have a large initial pool of follicles, having a low risk for early ovarian aging.

A particular case of ovarian aging is represented by women with premature ovarian failure (POF), representing 20% of infertile population. These patients associate with an increased risk of miscarriages [106] and a poor response to ovarian stimulation. POF refers to women with ovarian insufficiency before the age of 40. The genetic and autoimmune factors are the most important causes of POF. POF could appear also iatrogenic after surgery or chemotherapy [107].

Ovarian aging is accompanied by endometrial aging. The old endometrium is still responsive to ovarian steroids and is characterized by increase in collagen content, a reduced number of stromal cells, reduced tissue deoxyribonucleic acid contents, and fewer estrogen receptors on endometrial cells. There is significant evidence that aging endometrium is a major determinant of reduced fecundity, where age and aging ovaries are the major determinant of higher abortion rate with age. In women older than 35 years, endometrial biopsy shows delayed or absent secretory maturation which determines implantation failure. However, IVF donor programs show satisfactory pregnancy rates in older women; therefore, from the reproductive point of view, the aging ovary is more important than the aging endometrium.

4. Conclusions

The inexorable effect of age on ovarian function is well known with a gradual decline in fertility by the age of 40, followed by an abrupt decrease thereafter and a cessation of ovarian function at menopause. The impact of age is not only due to a decreased number but also due to a decrease in quality of the oocytes, resulting in a high rate of chromosomal aneuploidy and a reduced implantation rate. The main mechanism assumed to be involved in ovarian aging is a reduced defense against oxidative stress, ROS, and RCS accumulation which damage the ovarian compartments, generating shortening of the telomeres and mitochondrial dysfunction.

On the other hand, in men, the semen quality and testicular function were found to gradually decrease with age, and most of the studies also describe a negative impact on fertility. The mechanisms underlying decreased fertility are genetic (chromosomal aneuploidies, DNA mutations) and epigenetics changes. However, whether these effects of aging in men can be overcome by assisted reproductive technologies is not clear yet as the results of the studies are inconsistent.

Author details

Alice Ioana Albu* and Dragos Albu

*Address all correspondence to: albualice@yahoo.com

Carol Davila University of Medicine and Pharmacy, Bucharest, Romania

References

[1] Bray I, Gunnell D, Davey SG. Advanced paternal age: How old is too old? Journal of Epidemiology and Community Health. 2006;**60:**851-853

[2] Office for National Statistics. Birth Statistics: Review of the Registrar General on Births and Family Building Patterns in England and Wales. London: Stationery Office; 2002

[3] Olsen J. Subfecundity according to the age of the mother and the father. Danish Medical Bulletin. 1990;**37**:281-282

[4] Joffe M, Li Z. Male and female factors in fertility. American Journal of Epidemiology. 1994;**140**(10):921-929

[5] Sallmen M, Luukkonen R. Is the observed association between increasing paternal age and delayed conception an artefact? Human Reproduction. 2001;**16**:2027-2028

[6] de La Rochebrochard E, Thonneau P. Paternal age or 1⁄440 years: An important risk factor for infertility. American Journal of Obstetrics and Gynecology. 2003;**189**:901-905

[7] Hassan MA, Killick SR. Effect of male age on fertility: Evidence for the decline in male fertility with increasing age. Fertility and Sterility. 2003;**79**:1520-1527

[8] Araujo AB, Mohr BA, McKinlay JB. Changes in sexual function in middle-aged and older men: Longitudinal data from the Massachusetts Male Aging Study. Journal of the American Geriatrics Society. 2004;**52**:1502-1509

[9] Dunson DB, Baird DD, Colombo B. Increased infertility with age in men and women. Obstetrics & Gynecology. 2004;**103**:51-56

[10] Wu FCW, Tajar A, Pye SR, Silman AJ, Finn JD, O'Neill TW, Bartfai G, Casanueva F, Forti G, Giwercman A, et al. Hypothalamic-pituitary-testicular axis disruptions in older men are differentially linked to age and modifiable risk factors: The European Male Aging Study. Journal of Clinical Endocrinology and Metabolism. 2008;**93**:2737-2745

[11] Kaufman JM, Vermeulen A. The decline of androgen levels in elderly men and its clinical and therapeutic implications. Endocrine Reviews. 2005;**26**:833-876

[12] Harman SM, Metter EJ, Tobin JD, Pearson J, Blackman MR. Longitudinal effects of aging on serum total and free testosterone levels in healthy men. Journal of Clinical Endocrinology and Metabolism. 2001;**86**:724-731

[13] Feldman HA, Longcope C, Derby CA, Johannes CB, Araujo AB, Coviello AD, Bremner WJ, McKinlay JB. Age trends in the level of serum testosterone and other hormones in middle-aged men: Longitudinal results from the Massachusetts Male Aging Study. Journal of Clinical Endocrinology and Metabolism. 2002;**87**:589-598

[14] Derby CA, Zilber S, Brambilla D, Morales KH, McKinlay JB. Body mass index, waist circumference and waist to hip ratio and change in sex steroid hormones: The Massachusetts Male Ageing Study. Clinical Endocrinology. 2006;**65**:125-131

[15] Mohr BA, Bhasin S, Link CL, O'Donnell AB, McKinlay JB. The effect of changes in adiposity on testosterone levels in older men: Longitudinal results from the Massachusetts Male Aging Study. European Journal of Endocrinology. 2006;**155**:443-452

[16] Travison TG, Araujo AB, Kupelian V, O'Donnell AB, McKinlay JB. The relative contributions of aging, health, and lifestyle factors to serum testosterone decline in men. Journal of Clinical Endocrinology and Metabolism. 2007;**92**:549-555

[17] Lapauw B, Goemaere S, Zmierczak H, Van Pottelbergh I, Mahmoud A, Taes Y, De Bacquer D, Vansteelandt S, Kaufman JM. The decline of serum testosterone levels in community-dwelling men over 70 years of age: Descriptive data and predictors of longitudinal changes. European Journal of Endocrinology. 2008;**159**:459-468

[18] Camacho EM, Huhtaniemi IT, O'Neill TW, Finn JD, Pye SR, Lee DM, Tajar A, Bartfai G, Boonen S, Casanueva FF, Forti G, Giwercman A, Han TS, Kula K, Keevil B, Lean ME, Pendleton N, Punab M, Vanderschueren D, Wu FC, The EMAS Group. Age-associated changes in hypothalamic-pituitary-testicular function in middle-aged and older men are modified by weight change and lifestyle factors: Longitudinal results from the European Male Ageing Study. European Journal of Endocrinology. 2013;**168**:445-455

[19] Wu FC, Tajar A, Beynon JM, et al. Identification of late-onset hypogonadism in middle-aged and elderly men. New England Journal of Medicine. 2010;**363**:123-135

[20] Neaves WB, Johnson L, Porter JC, Parker Jr CR, Petty CS. Leydig cell numbers, daily sperm production, and serum gonadotropin levels in aging men. Journal of Clinical Endocrinology and Metabolism. 1984;**59**:756-763

[21] Veldhuis JD, Veldhuis NJ, Keenan DM, Iranmanesh A. Age diminishes the testicular steroidogenic response to repeated intravenous pulses of recombinant human LH during acute GnRH-receptor blockade in healthy men. American Journal of Physiology Endocrinology and Metabolism. 2005 Apr;**288**(4):E775-E781. [Epub: November 30, 2004]

[22] Winters SJ, Wang C, Fortigel Study Group. LH and non-SHBG testosterone and estradiol levels during testosterone replacement of hypogonadal men: Further evidence that steroid negative feedback increases as men grow older. Journal of Andrology. 2010 May-Jun;**31**(3):281-287. DOI: 10.2164/jandrol.109.009035. [Epub: December 3, 2009]

[23] Huhtaniemi IT, Pye SR, Holliday KL, Thomson W, O'Neill TW, Platt H, Payne D, John SL, Jiang M, Bartfai G, Boonen S, Casanueva FF, Finn JD, Forti G, Giwercman A, Han TS, Kula K, Lean ME, Pendleton N, Punab M, Silman AJ, Vanderschueren D, Labrie F, Wu FC, European Male Aging Study Group. Effect of polymorphisms in selected genes involved in pituitary-testicular function on reproductive hormones and phenotype in aging men. Journal of Clinical Endocrinology and Metabolism. 2010 Apr;**95**(4):1898-1908. DOI: 10.1210/jc.2009-2071. [Epub: February 19, 2010]

[24] Rolf C, Behre HM, Nieschlag E. Reproductive parameters of older compared to younger men of infertile couples. International Journal of Andrology. 1996 Jun;**19**(3):135-142

[25] Andolz P, Bielsa MA, Vila J. Evolution of semen quality in North-Eastern Spain: A study in 22,759 infertile men over a 36 year period. Human Reproduction. 1999 Mar;**14**(3):731-735

[26] Auger J, Kunstmann JM, Czyglik F, Jouannet P. Decline in semen quality among fertile men in Paris during the past 20 years. New England Journal of Medicine. 1995 Feb 2;**332**(5):281-285

[27] Schwartz D, Mayaux MJ, Spria A, Moscato ML, Jouannet P, Czyglik F, David G. Semen characteristics as a function of age in 833 fertile men. Fertility and Sterility. 1983;**39**:530-535

[28] Fisch H, Goluboff ET, Olson JH, Feldshuh J, Broder SJ, Barad DH. Semen analysis in 1,283 men from the United States over a 25-year period: No decline in quality. Fertility and Sterility. 1996;**65**:1009-1014

[29] Rolf C, Kenkel S, Nieschlag E. Age-related disease pattern in infertile men: Increasing incidence of infections in older patients. Andrologia. 2002;**34**:209-217. DOI: 10.1046/j.1439-0272.2002.00505.x

[30] Brahem S, Mehdi M, Elghezal H, Saad A. The effects of male aging on semen quality, sperm DNA fragmentation and chromosomal abnormalities in an infertile population. Journal of Assisted Reproduction and Genetics. 2011 May;**28**(5):425-432. DOI: 10.1007/s10815-011-9537-5. [Epub: February 3, 2011]

[31] Petersen PM, Seierøe K, Pakkenberg B. The total number of Leydig and Sertoli cells in the testes of men across various age groups—a stereological study. Journal of Anatomy. 2015 Feb;**226**(2):175-179. DOI: 10.1111/joa.12261. [Epub: December 25, 2014]

[32] Jiang H, Zhu WJ, Li J, Chen QJ, Liang WB, Gu YQ. Quantitative histological analysis and ultrastructure of the aging human testis. International Urology and Nephrology. 2014 May;**46**(5):879-885. DOI: 10.1007/s11255-013-0610-0. [Epub: November 26, 2013]

[33] Sartorius GA, Nieschlag E. Paternal age and reproduction. Human Reproduction. 2010;**16**(1):65-79

[34] Johnson SL, Dunleavy J, Gemmell NJ, Nakagawa S. Consistent age-dependent declines in human semen quality: A systematic review and meta-analysis. Ageing Research Reviews. 2015;**19**:22-33

[35] Moskovtsev SI, Willis J, Mullen JB. Age-related decline in sperm deoxyribonucleic acid integrity in patients evaluated for male infertility. Fertility and Sterility. 2006;**85**:496-499

[36] Singh NP, Muller CH, Berger RE. Effects of age on DNA double-strand breaks and apoptosis in human sperm. Fertility and Sterility. 2003;**80**:1420-1430

[37] Spano M, Bonde JP, Hjollund HI, Kolstad HA, Cordelli E, Leter G. Sperm chromatin damage impairs human fertility. The Danish First Pregnancy Planner Study Team. Fertility and Sterility. 2000;**73**:43-50

[38] Giwercman A, Lindstedt L, Larsson M, Bungum M, Spano M, Levine RJ, et al. Sperm chromatin structure assay as an independent predictor of fertility in vivo: A case-control study. International Journal of Andrology. 2010;**33**:e221-e227

[39] Loft S, Kold-Jensen T, Hjollund NH, Giwercman A, Gyllemborg J, Ernst E, et al. Oxidative DNA damage in human sperm influences time to pregnancy. Human Reproduction. 2003;**18**:1265-1272

[40] Zini A. Are sperm chromatin and DNA defects relevant in the clinic? Systems Biology in Reproductive Medicine. 2011;**57**:78-85

[41] Bungum M, Humaidan P, Axmon A, Spano M, Bungum L, Erenpreiss J, et al. Sperm DNA integrity assessment in prediction of assisted reproduction technology outcome. Human Reproduction. 2007;**22**:174-179

[42] Collins JA, Barnhart KT, Schlegel PN. Do sperm DNA integrity tests predict pregnancy with in vitro fertilization? Fertility and Sterility. 2008;**89**:823-831

[43] Practice Committee of the American Society for Reproductive Medicine. The clinical utility of sperm DNA integrity testing: A guideline. Fertility and Sterility. 2013;**99**:673-677

[44] Robinson L, Gallos ID, Conner SJ, Rajkhowa M, Miller D, Lewis S, et al. The effect of sperm DNA fragmentation on miscarriage rates: A systematic review and meta-analysis. Human Reproduction. 2012;**27**:2908-2917

[45] Frattarelli JL, Miller KA, Miller BT, Elkind-Hirsch K, Scott Jr RT. Male age negatively impacts embryo development and reproductive outcome in donor oocyte assisted reproductive technology cycles. Fertility and Sterility. 2008;**90**:97-103

[46] Wdowiak A, Bakalczuk S, Bakalczuk G. The effect of sperm DNA fragmentation on the dynamics of the embryonic development in intracytoplasmatic sperm injection. Reproductive Biology. 2015 Jun;**15**(2):94-100. DOI: 10.1016/j.repbio.2015.03.003. [Epub: April 2, 2015]

[47] Simon L, Murphy K, Shamsi MB, Liu L, Emery B, Aston KI. Paternal influence of sperm DNA integrity on early embryonic development. Human Reproduction. 2014;**29**:2402-2412

[48] Borini A, Tarozzi N, Bizzaro D, Bonu MA, Fava L, Flamigni C, Coticchio G. Sperm DNA fragmentation: Paternal effect on early post-implantation embryo development in ART. Human Reproduction. 2006 Nov;**21**(11):2876-2881. [Epub: June 22, 2006]

[49] Sivanarayana T, Krishna ChR, Prakash GJ, Krishna KM, Madan K, Rani BS, Sudhakar G, Raju GA. CASA derived human sperm abnormalities: Correlation with chromatin packing and DNA fragmentation. Journal of Assisted Reproduction and Genetics. 2012 Dec;**29**(12):1327-1334. DOI: 10.1007/s10815-012-9885-9. [Epub: November 8, 2012]

[50] Martin RH. Meiotic errors in human oogenesis and spermatogenesis. Reproductive BioMedicine Online. 2008 Apr;**16**(4):523-531

[51] Griffin DK, Abruzzo MA, Millie EA, Sheean LA, Feingold E, Sherman SL, Hassold TJ. Non-disjunction in human sperm: Evidence for an effect of increasing paternal age. Human Molecular Genetics. 1995;**4**:2227-2232

[52] Sharma R, Agarwal A, Rohra VK, Assidi M, Abu-Elmagd M, Turki RF. Effects of increased paternal age on sperm quality, reproductive outcome and associated epigenetic risks to offspring. Reproductive Biology and Endocrinology. 2015;**13**:35. DOI: 10.1186/s12958-015-0028-x

[53] Bosch M, Rajmil O, Egozcue J, Templado C. Linear increase of structural and numerical chromosome 9 abnormalities in human sperm regarding age. European Journal of Human Genetics. 2003 Oct;**11**(10):754-759

[54] Fonseka KG, Griffin DK. Is there a paternal age effect for aneuploidy? Cytogenetic and Genome Research. 2011;**133**(2-4):280-291. DOI: 10.1159/000322816. [Epub: January 6, 2011]

[55] Dakouane-Giudicelli M, Bicchieray L, Bergere M, Albert M, Vialard F, Selva J. A histomorphometric and cytogenetic study of testis from men 29-102 years old. Fertility and Sterility. 2005 Apr;**83**(4):923-928

[56] Brinkworth MH, Schmid TE. Effect of age on testicular germ cell apoptosis and sperm aneuploidy in MF-1 mice. Teratogenesis, Carcinogenesis, and Mutagenesis. 2003;(Suppl 2): 103-109

[57] De Souza E, Morris JK, EUROCAT Working Group. Collaborators. Case-control analysis of paternal age and trisomic anomalies. Archives of Disease in Childhood. 2010 Nov;**95**(11):893-897. DOI: 10.1136/adc.2009.176438. [Epub: June 28, 2010]

[58] Arnedo N, Templado C, Sánchez-Blanque Y, Rajmil O, Nogués C. Sperm aneuploidy in fathers of Klinefelter's syndrome offspring assessed by multicolour fluorescent in situ hybridization using probes for chromosomes 6, 13, 18, 21, 22, X and Y. Human Reproduction. 2006 Feb;**21**(2):524-528. [Epub: September 30, 2005]

[59] Steiner B, Masood R, Rufibach K, Niedrist D, Kundert O, Riegel M, Schinzel A. An unexpected finding: Younger fathers have a higher risk for offspring with chromosomal aneuploidies. European Journal of Human Genetics. 2015 Apr;**23**(4):466-472. DOI: 10.1038/ejhg.2014.122. [Epub: July 9, 2014]

[60] Fisch H, Hyun G, Golden R, Hensle TW, Olsson CA, Liberson GL. The influence of paternal age on Down syndrome. Journal of Urology. 2003;**169**:2275-2278

[61] Hassold T, Sherman S. Down syndrome: Genetic recombination and the origin of the extra chromosome 21. Clinical Genetics. 2000;**57**:95-100

[62] Hatch M, Kline J, Levin B, Hutzler M, Warburton D. Paternal age and trisomy among spontaneous abortions. Human Genetics. 1990;**85**:355-361

[63] Naguib KK, Al-Awadi SA, Moussa MA, Bastaki L, Gouda S, Redha MA, Mustafa F, Tayel SM, Abulhassan SA, Murthy DS. Trisomy 18 in Kuwait. International Journal of Epidemiology. 1999;**28**:711-716

[64] Archer NP, Langlois PH, Suarez L, Brender J, Shanmugam R. Association of paternal age with prevalence of selected birth defects. Birth Defects Research Part A: Clinical and Molecular Teratology. 2007;**79**:27-34

[65] García-Ferreyra J, Luna D, Villegas L, Romero R, Zavala P, Hilario R, Dueñas-Chacón J. High aneuploidy rates observed in embryos derived from donated oocytes are related to male aging and high percentages of sperm DNA fragmentation. Clinical Medicine Insights: Reproductive Health. 2015 Nov 11;**9**:21-27. DOI: 10.4137/CMRH.S32769. [eCollection 2015]

[66] Crow JF. The origins, patterns and implications of human spontaneous mutation. Nature Reviews Genetics. 2000;**1**:40-47

[67] Kong A, Frigge ML, Masson G, Besenbacher S, Sulem P, Magnusson G, et al. Rate of de novo mutations and the importance of father's age to disease risk. Nature. 2012;**488**: 471-475

[68] Martien S, Abbadie C. Acquisition of oxidative DNA damage during senescence: The first step toward carcinogenesis? Annals of the New York Academy of Sciences. 2007;**1119**:51-63

[69] Kimura M, Cherkas LF, Kato BS, Demissie S, Hjelmborg JB, Brimacombe M, Cupples A, Hunkin JL, Gardner JP, Lu X, Cao X, Sastrasinh M, Province MA, Hunt SC, Christensen K, Levy D, Spector TD, Aviv A. Offspring's leukocyte telomere length, paternal age, and telomere elongation in sperm. PLoS Genetics. 2008 Feb;**4**(2):e37. DOI: 10.1371/journal.pgen.0040037

[70] Aviv A, Susser E. Leukocyte telomere length and the father's age enigma: Implications for population health and for life course. International Journal of Epidemiology. 2013 Apr;**42**(2):457-462. DOI: 10.1093/ije/dys236. [Published online: February 4, 2013]

[71] Wright WE, Piatyszek MA, Rainey WE, Byrd W, Shay JW. Telomerase activity in human germline and embryonic tissues and cells. Developmental Genetics. 1996;**18**(2):173-179

[72] Aston KI, Hunt SC, Susser E, et al. Divergence of sperm and leukocyte age-dependent telomere dynamics: Implications for male-driven evolution of telomere length in humans. Molecular Human Reproduction. 2012;**18**:517-522

[73] Ferlin A, Rampazzo E, Rocca MS, Keppel S, Frigo AC, De Rossi A, Foresta C. In young men sperm telomere length is related to sperm number and parental age. Human Reproduction. 2013 Dec;**28**(12):3370-3376. DOI: 10.1093/humrep/det392. [Epub: October 27, 2013]

[74] Thilagavathi J, Venkatesh S, Dada R. Telomeres length in reproduction. Andrologia. 2013 Oct;**45**(5):289-304

[75] Antunes DM, Kalmbach KH, Wang F, Dracxler RC, Seth-Smith ML, Kramer Y, Buldo-Licciardi J, Kohlrausch FB, Keefe DL. A single-cell assay for telomere DNA content shows increasing telomere length heterogeneity, as well as increasing mean telomere length in human spermatozoa with advancing age. Journal of Assisted Reproduction and Genetics. 2015 Nov;**32**(11):1685-1690. DOI: 10.1007/s10815-015-0574-3. [Epub: September 28, 2015]

[76] Allsopp RC, Vaziri H, Patterson C, Goldstein S, Younglai EV, Futcher AB, Greider CW, Harley CB. Telomere length predicts replicative capacity of human fibroblasts. Proceedings of the National Academy of Sciences of the United States of America. 1992;**89**:10114-10118

[77] Oakes CC, Smiraglia DJ, Plass C, Trasler JM, Robaire B. Aging results in hypermethylation of ribosomal DNA in sperm and liver of male rats. Proceedings of the National Academy of Sciences of the United States of America. 2003;**100**:1775-1780

[78] Bloom DE. 7 billion and counting. Science. 2011;**333**:562-569

[79] Menken J, Trussell J, Larsen U. Age and infertility. Science. 1986;**233**:1389-1394

[80] Gray RH, Wu LY. Subfertility and risk of spontaneous abortion. American Journal of Public Health. 2000;**90:**1432-1434

[81] Gleicher N. Ovarian aging: Is there a "norm"? Contemporary Obstetrics and Gynaecology. 2005;**50**:65-75

[82] Faddy MJ, Gosden RG. A model conforming the decline in follicle numbers to the age of menopause in women. Human Reproduction. 1996;**11**:1484-1486

[83] Faddy MJ, Gosden RG. A mathematical model of follicle dynamics in the human ovary. Human Reproduction. 1995;**10**:770-775

[84] Gleicher N, Weghofer A, Barad D. Female infertility due to abnormal autoimmunity: Frequently overlooked and greatly underappreciated. Part I. Expert Review of Obstetrics & Gynecology. 2007;**2**:453-464

[85] Gleicher N, Weghofer A, Barad D. Female infertility due to abnormal autoimmunity: Frequently overlooked and greatly underappreciated. Part II. Expert Review of Obstetrics & Gynecology. 2007;**2**:465-475

[86] Feuerstein P, Puard V, Chevalier C, Teusan R, Cadoret V, Guerif F, et al. Genomic assessment of human cumulus cell marker genes as predictors of oocyte developmental competence: Impact of various experimental factors. PLoS One. 2012;**7**:e40449

[87] Tatone C, Amicarelli F. The aging ovary—the poor granulosa cells. Fertility and Sterility. 2013;**99**:12-17

[88] Hardy R, Kuh D. Reproductive characteristics and the age at inception of the perimenopause in a British National Cohort. American Journal of Epidemiology. 1999;**149**:612-620

[89] Faddy MJ. Follicle dynamics during ovarian aging. Molecular and Cellular Endocrinology. 2000 May;**163**(1-2):43-48

[90] Gleicher N, Barad DH. The aging ovary. In: Deligdisch L, Kase NG, Cohen CJ, eds. Altchek's Diagnosis and Management of Ovarian Disorders. 3rd ed. Cambridge: Cambridge University Press; 2013:275-286. DOI:10.1017/CBO9781139003254.020

[91] Kalmbach KH, Fontes Antunes DM, Dracxler RC, Knier TW, Seth-Smith ML, Wang F, Liu L, Keefe DL. Telomeres and human reproduction. Fertility and Sterility. 2013 Jan;**99**(1):23-29. DOI: 10.1016/j.fertnstert.2012.11.039

[92] Liu L, Franco S, Spyropoulos B, Moens PB, Blasco MA, Keefe DL. Irregular telomeres impair meiotic synapsis and recombination in mice. Proceedings of the National Academy of Sciences of the United States of America. 2004 Apr 27;**101**(17):6496-6501

[93] Liu L, Blasco MA, Keefe DL. Requirement of functional telomeres for metaphase chromosome alignments and integrity of meiotic spindles. EMBO Reports. 2002 Mar;**3**(3):230-234

[94] Keefe DL, Liu L, Marquard K. Telomeres and aging-related meiotic dysfunction in women. Cellular and Molecular Life Sciences. 2007 Jan;**64**(2):139-143

[95] Agarwal A, Aponte-Mellado A, Premkumar BJ, Shaman A, Gupta S. The effects of oxidative stress on female reproduction: A review. Reproductive Biology and Endocrinology. 2012;**10**:49

[96] Harman D. Aging: A theory based on free radical and radiation chemistry. Journal of Gerontology. 1956;**11**:298-300

[97] Lim J, Luderer U. Oxidative damage increases and antioxidant gene expression decreases with aging in the mouse ovary. Biology of Reproduction. 2011;**84**:775-782

[98] Ito M, Muraki M, Takahashi Y, Imai M, Tsukui T, Yamakawa N, et al. Glutathione S-transferase theta 1 expressed in granulosa cells as a biomarker for oocyte quality in age-related infertility. Fertility and Sterility. 2008;**90**:1026-1035

[99] Ito M, Imai M, Muraki M, Miyado K, Qin J, Kyuwa S, et al. GSTT1 is upregulated by oxidative stress through p38-MK2 signaling pathway in human granulosa cells: Possible association with mitochondrial activity. Aging. 2011;**3**:1213-1223

[100] Mano J. Reactive carbonyl species: Their production from lipid peroxides, action in environmental stress, and the detoxification mechanism. Plant Physiology and Biochemistry. 2012;**59**: 90-97

[101] Goldin A, Beckman JA, Schmidt AM, Creager MA. Advanced glycation end products: Sparking the development of diabetic vascular injury. Circulation. 2006;**114**:597-605

[102] Fujii EY, Nakayama M. The measurements of RAGE, VEGF, and AGEs in the plasma and follicular fluid of reproductive women: The influence of aging. Fertility and Sterility. 2010;**94**:694-700

[103] Yeh J, Kim BS, Peresie J. Ovarian vascular endothelial growth factor and vascular endothelial growth factor receptor patterns in reproductive aging. Fertility and Sterility. 2008;**89**:1546-1556

[104] Sato T, Iwaki M, Shimogaito N, Wu X, Yamagishi S, Takeuchi M. TAGE (toxic AGEs) theory in diabetic complications. Current Molecular Medicine. 2006;**6**:351-358

[105] Gleicher N, Weghofer A, Oktay K, Barad D. Can the FMR1 (fragile X) gene serve as predictor of response to ovarian stimulation? Reproductive Sciences. 2008 Feb;**16**(5):462-467. DOI: 10.1177/1933719108328617

[106] Chand AL, Robertson DM, Shelling AN, Harrison CA. Mutational analysis of betaglycan/TGF-betaRill in premature ovarian failure. Fertility and Sterility. 2007;**87**:210-212

[107] Dixit H, Rao KL, Padmalatha VV, Kanakavalli M, Deenadayal M, Gupta N, Chakrabarty BN, Singh L. Mutational analysis of the betaglycan gene-coding region in susceptibility for ovarian failure. Human Reproduction. 2006;**21**:2041-2046

Chapter 3

Diagnosis, Pathogenesis and Management of Polycystic Ovary Syndrome

Fan Wang and Zhengchao Wang

Additional information is available at the end of the chapter

http://dx.doi.org/10.5772/67877

Abstract

Polycystic ovary syndrome (PCOS) is one of the most common reproductive endocrine diseases occurs among women of childbearing age, which is affected by many factors, but its precise pathophysiology has not yet been determined. The heterogeneous of PCOS is reflected in its complex endocrine dysfunction of the hypothalamic-pituitary-gonadal axis (HPG axis) and its multiple clinical features, such as obesity, insulin resistance, hyperandrogenism and anovulation. Meanwhile, women with PCOS also have an increased risk of major cardiovascular events, most notably type 2 diabetes, cardiovascular disease and atherosclerosis. So far, many therapies are available for improving reproductive and metabolic abnormalities in PCOS patients, in which lifestyle modification and insulin-sensitizing agents are more effective management strategies.

Keywords: polycystic ovary syndrome, hypothalamic-pituitary-gonadal axis, obesity, insulin resistance, hyperandrogenism

1. Introduction

Polycystic ovary syndrome (PCOS) is a prevalent heterogeneous disorder linked with disturbances of reproductive, endocrine and metabolic function [1], which is characterized by insulin resistance (IR), androgen excess and ovarian dysfunction and can increase the occurrence of the risks of other diseases, but its precise pathophysiology has not yet been determined. Recent years, much more studies showed that neuroendocrine dysfunction plays an important role in the pathophysiology of PCOS [9]. In PCOS, there are complex interactions between abnormal ovarian steroidogenesis, hyperinsulinemia and endocrine dysfunction of the hypothalamic-pituitary-gonadal axis (HPG axis) [2, 3]. HPG axis plays a crucial regulatory role in various life activities in mammal and consists of a complex network of hypothalamic neurons of gonadotropin releasing hormone (GnRH) and pituitary gonadotropin (GnRH) neurons capable of gonadotropic hormone (GH) and their target organs [4], in which hypothalamic-pituitary-adrenal axis (HPA) and hypothalamic-pituitary-ovarian axis (HPO) in the female reproductive system play a vital effect. Recent studies have found that the role of HPA and HPO axis in PCOS endocrine dysfunction, such as abnormal GnRH pulse frequency, increased LH/FSH ratio, adrenal and ovarian excess androgens [1].

PCOS patients with obesity, insulin resistance (IR), hyperandrogenism, are important pathogenic factors for the metabolic abnormalities [5]. PCOS not only can affect the female reproductive function, but also increase the incidence risk of tumors such as endometrial cancer, type 2 diabetes and cardiovascular disease [6]. PCOS is closely related to metabolic syndrome. The metabolic syndrome is significantly increased in PCOS patients; moreover, women with metabolic syndrome often suffer from PCOS, showed the related endocrine and metabolic characteristics [7] IR/compensatory hyperinsulinemia are, androgen excess/hyperandrogenism, the basic characteristics of metabolic abnormalities in PCOS patients. Obesity is recognized as the most common risk factor for IR. IR is not limited to the scope of glucose metabolism, lipid metabolism and vascular disease [5–7].

Weight loss is associated with metabolic syndrome, a key treatment of PCOS, including diet control and exercise [8]. Dietary options are low-fat foods, including the amount of protein, high carbohydrates, high fiber, whole grains, fruits, vegetables and so on. Lifestyle changes can reduce weight, even if a small part of body weight but can reduce the central distribution of fat and improve insulin sensitivity, plasma insulin levels and can also make obese patients to restore self-confidence, psychological healthy growth [9, 10]. Insulin sensitizing drugs (ISDs) not only reduce the role of obesity, but also have a good effect on obesity-induced endocrine disorders [10], and then much more studies demonstrated ISDs, such as metformin, thiazolidinediones(TZDs) and D-chiro-inositol, can improve some symptoms of PCOS patients, such as hyperandrogenism, anovulation and irregular menses [11].

2. Diagnostic criteria

PCOS was firstly described by Stein and Leventhal in 1935, which was the combination of oligo-ovulation and hyperandrogenism and accompanied by hirsutism, acne, and obesity [12, 13]. Over time, PCOS patients manifested a wide range of signs and symptoms, and there were no single diagnostic criteria in different regions or populations. So far, there are three recognized diagnostic criteria as following:

In 1990, the first formal diagnostic criteria for PCOS were come up by the National Institute of Child Health and Human Disease (NICHD), based on a majority opinion of the attendees, not clinical trial evidence. The NICHD criteria included (1) hyperandrogenism and/or hyperandrogenemia and (2) chronic anovulation. Both criteria must be present, and other diagnoses must be excluded to allow reaching a diagnosis of PCOS [14].

In 2003, a Rotterdam consensus workshop sponsored by the European Society of Human Reproduction and Embryology (ESHRE)/American Society of Reproductive Medicine (ASRM) revised the NIH diagnostic criteria according to clinical trials and familial studies. The revised criteria stated: (1) oligo- or anovulation, (2) hyperandrogenism and/or hyperandrogenemia, and (3) polycystic ovaries. PCOS remains a diagnosis of exclusion, but that two out of the following three criteria must be present. PCOS clinical manifestations may include: menstrual irregularities, signs of androgen excess, and obesity. Insulin resistance and elevated serum LH levels are also common features in PCOS [15].

In 2006, the American Androgen Excess Society (AES) and the PCOS Association systematically re-examined the key recognized features of PCOS based on the medical published literatures, the AE-PCOS criteria showed that (1) hyperandrogenism, including hirsutism and/or hyperandrogenism, (2) ovarian dysfunction, including oligo-anovulation and/or polycystic appearing ovaries, and (3) the exclusion of other androgen excess or related diseases. The AES criteria acknowledge that androgen excess is a necessary component of the diagnosis [16].

The diagnostic criteria must exclude other androgen excess diseases and ovulation dysfunctions and include androgen secreting neoplasms, Cushing's syndrome, 21-hydroxylase deficient congenital adrenal hyperplasia, thyroid disorders, hyperprolactinemia and premature ovarian failure [14–16].

3. Pathogenesis

3.1. HPA and HPO axis neuroendocrine dysfunction

3.1.1. Neuroendocrinology dysfunction of the hypothalamic-pituitary axis

In PCOS, the GnRH pulse frequency is increased to approximately one pulse per 50–60 min, and increases the total amount of GnRH [17], due to the increased endogenous GnRH response to LH. This GnRH secretion pattern leads to an increase in LH/FSH ratio [4]. The relative deficiency of FSH levels causes a decrease in aromatase activity in granulosa cells, leading to testosterone not aromatize into estrogen [18, 19]. Moreover, the ovarian sex hormones have feedback effects on the nervous system, affecting the secretion of gonadotropin and the frequency of GnRH pulse [18, 19]. Many studies have shown that low-dose E2 levels in PCOS long-term positive feedback to stimulate the hypothalamus and pituitary, leading to form high LH levels [18, 19]. Androgen in women with PCOS suppresses the negative feedback effect of progesterone on GnRH pulse frequency [20, 21].

3.1.2. Adrenal dysfunction

The type of androgen in normal women is mainly androstenedione (A2), testosterone (T), dehydroisoandrosterone (DHEA) and dehydroepiandrosterone sulfate (DHEAS). A2 and

T are mainly from the ovarian theca cell and luteal cell, while DHEA and DHEAS are almost from the adrenal gland [22]. About 20–30% of PCOS patients have the excess adrenal androgens, such as DHEAS, which influence the activity of P450c17α and increase the metabolism of peripheral cortisol, leading to the impaired negative feedback regulation of ACTH [23].

Early onset of adrenal function is characterized by the onset of early pubic and armpit hair and may continue to develop into PCOS, which is associated with elevated levels of DHEA, due to the CYP17A1 (P450c17α) dysfunction. Activation of CYP17A1 in the adrenal reticular region leads to an increase levels of DHEA [24]. A study has demonstrated the increased size of the adrenal reticular band and increased in normal adolescent P450c17α activity to increase the synthesis of DHEA, which is onset of premature adrenal function to the process of PCOS [25]. The adrenal androgens have feedback effect on increasing the hypothalamic secretion of LH, which, in turn, leads to increase the synthesis of ovarian androgen. Thus, the adrenal androgen may cause the changes of steroid synthesis in the ovary [26, 27].

3.1.3. Ovarian dysfunction

In fact, PCOS is the most common cause of anovulatory infertility, the morphological changes may be genetic, but ovulation or anovulation is mainly dependent on the follicular environment, may be due to excessive production of local endocrine factor [18, 28, 29]. Hyperandrogenism is one of the diagnostic criteria of PCOS, and ovarian hyperandrogenism can lead to excessive follicular atresia, follicular stasis and anovulation. In PCOS, the mechanism of ovarian androgen excess is mainly theca cells that are over-responsive to LH and excessively produced androgen [12, 13]. At the molecular level, cholesterol through a series of intermediate steps is converted to androgens in theca cell layer, and the disorganized regulation of androgen biosynthesis enzyme P450c17 results in hyperandrogenism [20, 21, 30].

In general, LH binds to its receptor to stimulate thecal cells to produce androstenedione and testosterone. In contrast, FSH mainly stimulates granulosa cells to aromatize these androgens into estrogens that is, two-cell theory [31]. In PCOS, the relative lack of FSH levels leads to a decrease in aromatase activity in granulosa cells, which prevents testosterone from converting into estrogen, while low-dose estrogen long term stimulates the hypothalamus and pituitary to form high LH levels by a positive feedback [18, 19]. Progesterone is a precursor of androgen and estrogen biosynthesis. Under the stimulation of LH, granulation cells luteinized after ovulation and increased the secretion of progesterone, but a decreased estrogen secretion promoted the failure to select the dominant follicle and accompanied by anovulation in PCOS rats and make granulosa cells could not be luteinized to reduce the serum progesterone concentration [2, 3].

In PCO, the disordered follicular development impacts oocyte development. In vitro fertilization studies found that PCOS patients have a lower oocyte implantation rate [32–34], due to oocytes which are exposed to high levels of androgens and other factors of abnormal levels, such as high insulin levels [3]. Gene chip analysis showed that abnormal endocrine and metabolic have a effects on the gene expression in PCOS oocyte, and most of the differentially expressed genes were upregulated in oocytes of PCOS patients [28, 29, 35].

3.2. Metabolic dysfunction

3.2.1. Androgen excess/hyperandrogenism

Hyperandrogenism is one of the most important endocrine features of PCOS [36]. Higher circulating androgen levels, on the one hand, can hinder the normal growth of follicles, resulting in oligoovulation or anovulation, which mainly manifests an abnormal menstrual cycle, usually oligomenorrhea/amenorrhea [36, 37], on the other hand, can cause hirsutism, acne, female hair loss and other clinical symptoms [38]. Many animal studies have shown that intrauterine androgen excess led to their offspring would be similar to the reproductive and metabolic characteristics of PCOS patients [39], and thus, androgen plays an important role in the pathogenesis of PCOS.

These clinical manifestations of hyperandrogenism will be obvious around puberty, due to both ovarian and adrenal androgens excess [40]. Excessive ovarian and adrenal gland secretion of androgens through the circulation transport into the peripheral adipose tissue and are aromatized into estrone [41]. Serum estrone excess continuously exerts feedback effects on the hypothalamus and pituitary, which manifests positive feedback effects on LH secretion and negative feedback effects of FSH secretion, leads to increase LH/FSH ratio. Low basal levels of FSH will be contribute to promote follicle development to a certain extent, but not mature, increased LH secretion, but no cyclical fluctuations, there are no LH peak, thus is the occurrence of oligoovulation, leading to infertility [1, 31]. In particular, androgen formation is also affected by insulin and insulin growth factor system, renin-angiotensin system (RAS), adiponectin, leptin, growth hormone and other factors.

Hirsutism can affect approximately 5–10% of reproductive-age women, while approximately 80% of hirsute patients will have PCOS. The increased activity of enzyme 5-α reductase in the hair follicle has elevated circulating testosterone and contributes to a dysregulation of hair follicle growth, which converts testosterone to dihydrotestosterone (DHT). Androgen excess increases hair follicle size, hair fiber diameter, and the proportion of time terminal hairs remains in the anagen (growth) phase [42].

3.2.2. Insulin resistance/hyperinsulinemia

In recent years, a large number of studies have established IR, obesity, hyperandrogenism and vascular endothelial dysfunction contribution to the occurrence and development of PCOS [43], IR can promote elevate serum insulin levels and increase the frequency of pulsatile GnRH secretion, cause elevated serum LH levels, and further promote excess androgen production [1]. The high levels of insulin result in the increased synthesis of androgen and inhibit the synthesis of sex hormone-binding globulin (SHBG) in liver, give rise to increase serum free androgen [44] and may induce the activity of insulin-like growth factor-1 and promote the synthesis of androgen [45]. Androgen can impact the growth and development of follicles, inhibit the formation of dominant follicles, and accumulate a large number of immature follicles, that is, the formation of the polycystic-like changes of the ovaries [46].

The interaction of insulin with its receptor results in dimerization of the receptor and facilitates recruitment and activation of downstream proteins via receptor autophosphorylation [47, 48]. Many physiological effects of insulin are mediated primarily via the phosphatidylinositol-3-kinase (PI3K) signaling pathway—metabolic effects and the mitogen-activated protein kinase (MAPK) signaling pathway—mitogenic effects [48]. Insulin no longer plays its metabolic role in insulin sensitive tissues, when insulin sensitivity is compromised in that insulin resistance occurs. When insulin insensitivity hinders glucose uptake in target tissue, insulin secretion is usually increased, leading to compensatory hyperinsulinemia [49].

Usually, the metabolic action of insulin is preferentially interfered, such as glucose uptake, while its mitogenic action can remain intact [47, 48]. In PCOS patients, insulin resistance impact on the synthesis, transport and degradation of glucose led to increase the blood glucose levels and serum insulin levels [50, 51]. At present, a large number of studies have found that PCOS patients with varying degrees of insulin resistance and compensatory hyperinsulinemia and in addition to systemic IR exist ovarian insulin resistance [52–54]. Much more studies have suggested that IR and hyperinsulinemia play an important role in the pathogenesis of PCOS [52]. IR and hyperinsulinemia are important features of chronic hyperandrogenic anovulatory women [52–54]. Therefore, PCOS is a syndrome as the combination of metabolism abnormalities and reproductive dysfunction.

3.2.3. *Obesity*

The development of obesity is a multifactorial and complex process, which can cause many changes in the endocrine system and thus damage to female reproductive function [55]. Obesity is one of the most common clinical manifestations of PCOS, and PCOS patients showed metabolic abnormalities that were independent of obesity and were generally associated with weight gain before menstruation or hyperandrogenism [56], thus suggesting the role of obesity in the progression of the pathogenesis of PCOS. Obesity is superimposed in PCOS, which is also associated with the hyperactivity of HPA, leading to increased adrenal androgen excess status [57]. Obese PCOS patients had lower SHBG levels than those with normal weight PCOS, which lead to translate into a higher circulating free testosterone [58]. Thus, there is a greater degree of hirsutism and menstrual disorders in obese PCOS women. It has been suggested that PCOS itself may cause weight gain [56]. More importantly, established superimposed obesity further promotes weight gain, which due to the deeper hyperinsulinism of obesity, exerts greater metabolic effects on insulin synthesis, leading to more rapid fat deposition [56].

PCOS is closely related to evaluate body fat distribution, especially abdominal fat [59, 60]. Most obese PCOS patients exhibit fat accumulation in the abdomen, especially in the viscera [59]. Abdominal obesity is strongly associated with the development of IR [59]. In particular, visceral adipose tissue is highly sensitive to lipolysis stimulated by androgens that will be contribute to the increased availability of free fatty acids (FFA) [60]. This, in turn, leads to induce the accumulation of hepatic fat, decreased hepatic insulin clearance and hepatic insulin resistance [61]. The fasting lipid profile of obese worsening PCOS is characterized by increased triglycerides and reduced HDL-C and may also reflect the effects of deeper degree of IR in obesity [62]. Increased circulating endothelin-1 and activation of the sympathetic nervous system and renin-angiotensin-aldosterone system are also contribution to worsening hypertension as a result of obesity in PCOS. Not surprisingly, most PCOS patients meeting the criteria of the metabolic syndrome are obese. In fact, abdominal obesity is the most common feature of metabolic syndrome in the disorder.

3.2.4. *Oxidative stress*

In recent years, effects of oxidative stress (OS) on the female reproductive system attract much more attention, such as superoxide dismutase (SOD), which are involved in the embryo implantation process, and follicular fluid antioxidant content will directly affect in vitro fertilization success rates [63–65].

Much more studies showed that the concentration levels of OS markers in PCOS higher than normal, such as lipid peroxidation (LPO) [66]. A study reported that the advanced oxidation protein products in women with PCOS were higher than that in health women with the same age and body mass index (BMI), while the total antioxidant levels were lower [67]. Previous studies suggested that OS is associated with obesity of PCOS patients, but recent studies have found elevated OS markers levels in lean PCOS patients [66].

IR is thought to be a cause of OS, which can lead to the occurrence of hyperglycemia, thus causes related cells to release reactive oxygen species (ROS), causing OS [68]. OS can damage cells and activate the expression of proinflammatory cytokines, which in turn promotes the occurrence of IR and hyperandrogenism [69]. The malondialdehyde (MDA) levels in PCOS patients with IR higher than PCOS patients without IR, but lower levels of peroxidase and zinc, which indicate high levels of OS in PCOS patients with IR [68–70]. Zinc is essential for the biological function of metalloproteinases, which not only participates in the synthesis, secretion, conduction and metabolism of insulin, and also with copper act on SOD and peroxidase (POD). Therefore, zinc deficiency may contribute to metabolic disorder in PCOS patients by affecting insulin function and reducing antioxidant content and may aggravate the degree of IR and the degree of antioxidant deficiency in PCOS patients [71].

OS markers in PCOS patients, such as MDA, thiol, and blood zinc, are associated with whose fertility, the levels of MDA in infertility PCOS patients higher than that in pregnant PCOS patients, while the MAD, sulfhydryl and blood zinc content are lower [67–71]. Therefore, eat more fruits and vegetables containing antioxidants, increased intake of vitamins, avoid drinking, smoking and intake of caffeine to maintain the balance between oxidants and antioxidants in the body, so as to maintain the health female reproductive system, which improving female fertility.

3.2.5. *Chronic low-grade inflammation*

Chronic low-grade inflammation is triggered an inflammatory response by nutrient metabolism excess, and its involved molecules and signaling pathways are similar to traditional inflammatory response, leading to the occurrence of some chronic metabolic diseases [72];

moreover, its related metabolic regulations are closely to reproductive function. Some complications of PCOS are closely associated with chronic low-grade inflammation, such as obesity, diabetes type 2 and cardiovascular disease, and inflammation factors may be responsible for long-term consequences of PCOS [73], such as C-reaction protein (CRP), tumor necrosis factor-α (TNF-α), interleukin-6 (IL-6), IL-18 and monocyte chemoattractant protein-1 (MCP-1). The first study demonstrating elevation of CRP in women with PCOS was carried out by Kelly, which suggested inflammation may be involved in occurrence and development of PCOS [74].

The inflammatory responses are induced by hyperlipidemia and IR, which not only lead to the occurrence and development of PCOS, and are also involved in the formation of long-term complications of PCOS. Some studies suggested that hyperandrogenism may be an inducing factor for chronic low-grade inflammation of PCOS [75], in turn the inflammatory responses further promote excessive ovarian androgen synthesis in PCOS patients [75]. In cellular level, inflammation upregulates the androgen biosynthesis enzyme CYP17 activity and thus promotes androgen synthesis [69]. Another study found that the stimulation of TNF-α increased the proliferation of androgen synthesis in rat interstitial cells, resulting in increased androgen secretion, which suggested that inflammation can further aggravate the performance of PCOS patients with hyperandrogenism [69, 74]. Interestingly, recent studies have found that hyperandrogenism may play an anti-inflammatory role in obese PCOS patients and demonstrated that the cycle effects of androgen were pleiotropic, and its role depends on whether obese individuals [60, 74].

Obesity increased PCOS patients with IR. IL-6, MCP-1 and TNF-α levels in patients with PCOS were significantly higher than those in controls, which were positively correlated with body weight and IR, suggesting that chronic low-grade inflammation in PCOS patients was closely related to obesity and IR [74]. Inflammatory signaling pathways interact with insulin signaling pathway, and macrophages were showed in adipose tissue of non-obese PCOS patients, which promoted the synthesis of inflammatory cytokines such as TNF-α and IL-6, which further led to the development of IR, which suggested that inflammatory may be responsible for IR in non-obese patients with PCOS [74].

Much more evidence shows PCOS patients with elevated inflammatory factors, suggesting that the body of patients in the inflammatory environment [76]. These inflammatory reactions in addition to the occurrence and development of PCOS can also cause type 2 diabetes, atherosclerosis, cardiovascular disease and other long-term complications. Therefore, the early administration of anti-inflammatory treatment may reduce the occurrence of the long-term complications of patients with PCOS.

3.2.6. Vitamin D deficiency

There are increasing evidences showed that vitamin D deficiency plays a major role in the in the pathogenesis of metabolic syndrome of PCOS [77]. Clinical studies have shown that type 2 diabetes and insulin resistance status are closely related to vitamin D deficiency [78]. In addition, studies have shown that vitamin D deficiency in patients has the increased risk of the long-term occurrence of hyperlipidemia and IR [78, 79], and in a prospective study of intervention, PCOS women with vitamin D supplementation, the secretion capacity of insulin was increased, and lipid levels were improved [80], suggesting the importance of vitamin D supplementation in treating patients with metabolic syndrome of the general population and PCOS population.

The correlation between vitamin D deficiency and PCOS is resulted from the deposition of 25-(OH) VD3 in adipose tissue [81]. The low level of 25-(OH) VD3 increases the risk of cancer, autoimmune diseases, diabetes and cardiovascular disease [82]. Much more researches showed that vitamin D deficiency ultimately leads to impaired insulin secretion, induces glucose intolerance, and reverses the vitamin D sufficient state [79–81]. Many studies showed that a low level of 25-(OH) VD3 was observed in type 2 diabetes, while it with insulin resistance and obesity are also confirmed in PCOS population [79–82]. So far, the mechanisms of low 25-(OH) VD3 levels and insulin resistance have not been well elucidated. First, 25-(OH) VD3 may stimulate insulin secretion by stimulating the expression of insulin receptors, thereby enhancing insulin responsiveness to glucose transport [79–82]. Second, 25-(OH) VD3 regulates intracellular and extracellular calcium ions levels, which is essential for insulin sensitive tissue such as skeletal muscle, adipose tissue mediated intracellular delivery of insulin. In addition, 25-(OH) VD3 deficiency may induce a hyperinflammatory response due to its role in regulating the immune system, which is also associated with IR [83].

A recent study confirms that high 25-(OH) VD3 levels in overweight and obese PCOS women are faster weight loss than that in women with low 25-(OH) VD3 levels due to better absorption of the low calorie diet, indicating that PCOS women with the high levels of 25-(OH) VD3, weight loss is one of the most effective treatments [84]. Therefore, vitamin D supplementation can be used as an adjunct to the treatment of PCOS.

4. PCOS management

4.1. Lifestyle changes

PCOS has become a social and psychological behavior disorder and a low risk factor for quality of life. In recent years, much more studies and treatment guidelines recommend that lifestyle intervention therapy is as a first-line treatment of PCOS [9].

Lifestyle intervention is mainly through diet and exercise methods [8, 9]. Diet therapy is mainly by controlling the total calorie intake of food, scientific and rational regulation of diet, in order to achieve the purpose of weight loss [8]. In addition to limiting calorie intake to achieve the purpose of weight loss can also be classified according to different macro nutrients, such as carbohydrates, protein and fat ratio [8]. The basic principle of exercise therapy is mainly through exercise to increase the consumption of glycogen and fat. Sports therapy is significantly able to achieve weight loss and also can enhance physical fitness. Studies have shown that women with cardiovascular disease, metabolic disorders, IR, overweight and obese can improve IR and reduce the risk of cardiovascular disease and abdominal fat by scientific, rational and regular exercise [85].

Lifestyle intervention achieves weight loss and long-term maintenance to reduce obesity for PCOS and directly improve the metabolic abnormalities, menstrual disorders, hairy acne and other symptoms [8]. A large number of studies have shown that weight loss in obese with PCOS patients, its symptoms can be improved to some extent. Low calorie diets, physical exercise and other lifestyle interventions, reduce 5–10% of body mass, can change or reduce menstrual disorders, hirsutism, acne and other symptoms, and increase the pregnancy rate, improve high blood lipids, high blood sugar IR and other symptoms and can reduce the incidence of miscarriage and cardiovascular disease.

4.2. Insulin sensitizing drugs

ISDs are used to control the hyperglycemia of type II diabetes. As time goes on, insulin resistance and compensatory hyperinsulinemia negatively affecting ovarian steroid biosynthesis and follicular recruitment and maturation were found in PCOS and play a critical role in its pathophysiology, and then, much more studies demonstrated that ISDs, such as metformin, thiazolidinediones (TZDs) and D-chiro-inositol, can improve some symptoms of PCOS patients, such as hyperandrogenism, anovulation and irregular menses [11].

Metformin is one of the most common ISDs to widely use in clinical treatment of PCOS, and as a biguanide can inhibit hepatic gluconeogenesis by affecting glucose metabolis and increase glucose uptake and reduce fatty acid oxidation in peripheral tissues, so as to achieve increasing insulin sensitivity [86, 87]. The effects of metformin on reproductive and on metabolic function of PCOS are mainly a reduction of circulating insulin levels. At the pituitary levels, hyperinsulinemia decreases SHBG synthesis, thus increasing circulating free androgens, at the muscular levels, it alters the mitochondrial oxidative metabolism, at the ovarian levels, hyperinsulinemia induces anovulation, follicular growth blockade and hyperandrogenism. Excess insulin increases the concentrations of androgen, which lead to block follicular maturation and increase cytochrome P450c17a activity [11, 86, 87]. On the other hand, metformin can improve the reproductive function at the HPO level. Insulin stimulates pituitary cells to modulate the normalize LH secretion pattern, thus hyperinsulinemia may be contribution to significantly decreasing LH plasma levels, then further impact ovarian function.

TZDs are peroxisome proliferator activating receptor γ (PPARγ) agonists, which are part of the superfamily of nuclear receptors are essential for adipocyte differentiation and growth, that in a lesser degree decrease hepatic glucose production, but more potently increase peripheral glucose uptake [87]. The metabolic effects of TZDs in PCOS are similar to metformin. Some mechanistic studies have shown that TZDS also decreases fasting glucose and insulin levels, AUCs for glucose and insulin levels, and glycosylated hemoglobin levels compared with placebo in women with PCOS, and troglitazone improves insulin-mediated glucose disposal as well as insulin-secretory defects in women with PCOS [86, 87].

D-Chiro-inositol, as a new insulin-sensitizing drug, has never been approved for clinical treatment in diabetes and PCOS but could improve insulin sensitivity by enhancing signal transduction via an alternative pathway for insulin action [87].

In a word, PCOS is usually diagnosed during the early reproductive years and still occurs in approximately 4–18% of reproductive-aged women. Although the pathophysiology of PCOS has yet not been clearly illuminated, there are much more related clinic manifestations had been deeper detected, which showed a number of its molecular mechanisms, and provided many new theoretical basis for clinical PCOS prevention and treatment.

Acknowledgements

This study was supported by National Natural Science Foundation of China (31271255), Fujian Provincial Natural Science Foundation (2016J01145) and Fujian Province Science and Technology Project of The Education Department (JAT160118 and JZ160426).

Author details

Fan Wang and Zhengchao Wang*

*Address all correspondence to: zcwang@fjnu.edu.cn

Provincial Key Laboratory for Developmental Biology and Neurosciences, College of Life Sciences, Fujian Normal University, Fuzhou, PR China

References

[1] Baskind NE, Balen AH. Hypothalamic-pituitary, ovarian and adrenal contributions to polycystic ovary syndrome. Best Practice & Research Clinical Obstetrics & Gynaecology, 2016;**37**:80-97. doi:10.1016/j.bpobgyn.2016.03.005

[2] Moore AM, Campbell RE. The neuroendocrine genesis of polycystic ovary syndrome: A role for arcuate nucleus GABA neurons. Journal of Steroid Biochemistry & Molecular Biology. 2016;**160**:106-117. doi:10.1016/j.jsbmb.2015.10.002

[3] Mantelli F, Moretti C, Macchi I, Massaro-Giordano G, Cozzupoli GM, Lambiase A, Bonini S. Effects of sex hormones on ocular surface epithelia: lessons learned from polycystic ovary syndrome. Journal of Cellular Physiology. 2016;**231**(5):971-975. doi:10.1002/jcp.25221

[4] Fan W, Kaizhuan X, Chaoji L,Zhengchao W. Regulation effects of PI3K signaling on HPG axis in mammalian. Chinese Journal of Cell Biology. 2013;**35**(7):1068-1072. doi:10.11844/cjcb.2013.07.0034

[5] Castelobranco C, Steinvarcel F, Osorio A, Ros C, Balasch J. Atherogenic metabolic profile in PCOS patients: Role of obesity and hyperandrogenism. Gynecological Endocrinology the Official Journal of the International Society of Gynecological Endocrinology. 2010;**26**:736. doi:10.3109/09513590.2010.481025

[6] Kousta E, Tolis G, Franks S. Polycystic ovary syndrome. Revised diagnostic criteria and long-term health consequences. Hormones. 2005;**4**:133.

[7] Teede HJ, Hutchison S, Zoungas S, Meyer C. Insulin resistance, the metabolic syndrome, diabetes, and cardiovascular disease risk in women with PCOS. Endocrine. 2006;**30**:45-53. doi:10.1385/ENDO:30:1:45

[8] Kirby MC, Effects of Dietary and Exercise Interventions On The Incidence of Metabolic Syndrome [thesis]. Jacksonville: University of North Florida; 2009.

[9] Moran LJ, Hutchison SK, Norman RJ, Teede HJ. Lifestyle changes in women with polycystic ovary syndrome. Cochrane Database of Systematic Reviews. 2011;**2**:CD007506. doi:10.1002/14651858.CD007506.pub3

[10] Curi DDG, Fonseca AM, Marcondes JAM, Almeida JA, Bagnoli VR, Soares JM Jr, Baracat EC. Metformin versus lifestyle changes in treating women with polycystic ovary syndrome. Gynecological Endocrinology: The Official Journal of the International Society of Gynecological Endocrinology. 2012;**28**:182-5. doi:10.3109/09513590.2011.583957

[11] Manguso F, Di Biase S, Falbo A, Giallauria F, Labella D, Tolino A, Lombardi G, Colao A, Palomba S. Metformin administration improves leukocyte count in women with polycystic ovary syndrome: A 6-month prospective study. European Journal of Endocrinology. 2007;**157**:69-73. doi:10.1530/EJE-07-0133

[12] Stein IF, Leventhal M. Amenorrhea associated with bilateral polycystic ovaries. American Journal of Obstetrics and Gynecology. 1935;**29**:181-191. doi:10.1016/S0002-9378(15)30642-6

[13] Azziz R, Adashi EY. Stein and Leventhal: 80 Years On. American Journal of Obstetrics & Gynecology. 2015;**214**:247.e1. doi:10.1016/j.ajog.2015.12.013

[14] Dewailly D. Diagnostic criteria for PCOS: need for a rethink? Best Practice & Research Clinical Obstetrics & Gynaecology, 2016;**3**:1-7. doi: 10.1016/j.bpobgyn.2016.03.009

[15] Group ESPCW. Revised 2003 consensus on diagnostic criteria and long-term health risks related to polycystic ovary syndrome (PCOS). Human Reproduction. 2004;**19**:19-25. doi:10.109/humrep/dch098

[16] Azziz R, Carmina E, Dewailly D, Diamanti-Kandarakis E, Escobar-Morreale HF, Futterweit W, Janssen OE, Legro RS, Norman RJ, Taylor AE, Witchel SF. The Androgen Excess and PCOS Society criteria for the polycystic ovary syndrome: The complete task force report. Fertility & Sterility. 2009;**91**:456-88. doi:10.1016/j.fertnstert.2008.06.035

[17] Pagan YL, Srouji SS, Jimenez Y, Emerson A, Gill S, Hall JE. Inverse relationship between luteinizing hormone and body mass index in polycystic ovary syndrome: investigation of hypothalamic and pituitary contributions. Journal of Clinical Endocrinology Metabolism. 2006;**91**:1309-16. doi:10.1210/jc.2005-2099

[18] Jones MR, Goodarzi MO. Genetic determinants of polycystic ovary syndrome: progress and future directions. Fertility & Sterility. 2016;**106**: 25-32. doi:10.1016/j.fertnstert.2016.04.040

[19] Woo I, Tobler K, Khafagy A, Christianson MS, Yates M, Garcia J. Predictive value of elevated LH/FSH ratio for ovulation induction in patients with polycystic ovary syndrome. Reproductive Sciences. 2015;**60**:495-500.

[20] Walters KA. Androgens in polycystic ovary syndrome: Lessons from experimental models. Current Opinion in Endocrinology, Diabetes & Obesity. 2016;**23**:257-263. doi:10.1097/MED.0000000000000245

[21] Luque-Ramírez M, Escobar-Morreale HF. Targets to treat androgen excess in polycystic ovary syndrome. Expert Opin Ther Targets. 2015;**19**:1545-1560. doi:10.1517/14728222.2015.1075511

[22] Allolio B, Arlt W. Dehydroepiandrosterone (DHEA) and androstenedione. European Journal of Haematology. 2012;**47**:313-5. doi:10.1017/CBO9781139003353.021

[23] Goodarzi MO, Enrico C, Ricardo A. DHEA, DHEAS and PCOS. Journal of Steroid Biochemistry & Molecular Biology. 2015;**145**:213-25. doi:10.1016/j.jsbmb.2014.06.003

[24] Abbott DH, Bird IM. Nonhuman primates as models for human adrenal androgen production: function and dysfunction. Reviews in Endocrine and Metabolic Disorders. 2009;**10**:33-42. doi:10.1007/s11154-008-9099-8

[25] Oberfield SE, Sopher AB, Gerken AT. Approach to the girl with early onset of pubic hair. Journal of Clinical Endocrinology & Metabolism. 2011;**96**:1610-22. doi:10.1210/jc.2011-0225

[26] Gonzalez F, Chang L, Horab T, Lobo RA. Evidence for heterogeneous etiologies of adrenal dysfunction in polycystic ovary syndrome. Fertility & Sterility. 1996;**66**:354-61. doi:10.1016/S0015-0282(16)58500-8

[27] Carmina E, Gonzalez F, Chang L, Lobo RA. Reassessment of adrenal androgen secretion in women with polycystic ovary syndrome. Obstetrics & Gynecology. 1995;**85**:971-6. doi:10.1016/0029-7844(95)00065-Y

[28] Azziz R. PCOS in 2015: New insights into the genetics of polycystic ovary syndrome. Nature Reviews Endocrinology. 2016;**12**:74-75. doi:10.1038/nrendo.2015.230

[29] Mahalingaiah S, Diamanti-Kandarakis E. Targets to treat metabolic syndrome in polycystic ovary syndrome. Expert Opinion on Therapeutic Targets. 2015;**19**:1561-1574. doi:10.1517/14728222.2015.1101067

[30] Vitek W, Hoeger K, Legro RS. Treatment strategies for infertile women with polycystic ovary syndrome. Minerva Ginecologica. 2016;**68**:450-457.

[31] Wang F, Zhang Z, Wang Z, Xiao K, Wang Q, Su J, Wang Z. Expression and clinical significance of the HIF-1a/ET-2 signaling pathway during the development and treatment of polycystic ovary syndrome. Journal of Molecular Histology. 2015;**46**:173-181. doi:10.1007/s10735-015-9609-4

[32] Mccartney CR, Marshall JC. Clinical practice. Polycystic ovary syndrome. New England Journal of Medicine. 2016;**375**:54-64. doi:10.1056/NEJMcp1514916

[33] Klein J, Craven M, Vuguin PM. Polycystic ovarian syndrome. Adolescent Medicine State of the Art Reviews. 2015;**26**(2):326-342.

[34] Shah D, Rasool S. Polycystic ovary syndrome and metabolic syndrome: The worrisome twosome? Climacteric. 2016;**19**(1):7-16. doi:10.3109/13697137.2015.1116505

[35] Rosenfield RL. The diagnosis of polycystic ovary syndrome in adolescents. Pediatrics. 2015;**136**(6):1154-1165. doi:10.1542/peds.2015-1430

[36] Ma L, Liu XM. Progress on treatment of PCOS with hyperandrogenism with traditional Chinese medicine. Global Traditional Chinese Medicine, 2012;**5**:633. doi:10.3969/j.issn:1674-1749.2012.08.024

[37] Mokhtar N, Lakany NE. The relationship between follicular fluid androgen concentrations and its receptor expression in granulosa cells from human follicles. Egyptian Journal of Biochemistry & Molecular Biology. 2013;**31**(1)

[38] Rutkowska A, Rachoń D. Bisphenol A (BPA) and its potential role in the pathogenesis of the polycystic ovary syndrome (PCOS). Gynecological Endocrinology: The Official Journal of the International Society of Gynecological Endocrinology. 2014;**30**:260-265. doi:10.3109/09513590.2013.871517

[39] Guerra MT, Sanabria M, Petrusz P, De Grava Kempinas W. Perinatal exposure to androgen excess and the effects on the rat uterine estradiol responsiveness. Environmental Toxicology. 2015;**31**:1460-1468. doi:10.1002/tox.22151

[40] Nader S. Hyperandrogenism during puberty in the development of polycystic ovary syndrome. Fertility & Sterility. 2013;**100**:39-42. doi:10.1016/j.fertnstert.2013.03.013

[41] Rodríguezgutiérrez R, Villarrealpérez JZ, Moralesmartinez FA, Rodríguez-Guajardo R, González-Saldivar G, Leonardo GMA, Alvarez-Villalobos N, Lavalle-Gonzalez FJ, González-González JG. Ovarian and adrenal androgens and their link to high human chorionic gonadotropin levels: A prospective controlled study. International Journal of Endocrinology, 2014;**2014**:191247.

[42] Cela E, Robertson C, Rush K, Kousta E, White DM, Wilson H, Kousta E, White DM, Wilson H, Lyons G, Kingsley P, McCarthy MI, Franks S. Prevalence of polycystic ovaries in women with androgenic alopecia. European Journal of Endocrinology. 2003;**149**:439-42. doi:10.1530/eje.0.1490439

[43] Yuan X, Hu T, Zhao H, Yuanyuan H, Rongcai Y, Jun L, Chuanhai Z, Hanlin Zhanga, Gang W, Huiqiao Z, Meng D, Jun Z, Haibin W, Qingsong L, Hyuek J L, Wanzhu J, ZiJiang C. Brown adipose tissue transplantation ameliorates polycystic ovary syndrome. Proceedings of the National Academy of Sciences of the United States of America. 2016;**113**:2708-2713. doi:10.1073/pnas.1523236113

[44] Laurent MR, Helsen C, Antonio L, Schollaert D, Joniau S, Vos MJ, Decallonne B, Hammond GL, Vanderschueren D, Claessens F. Effects of sex hormone-binding globulin (SHBG) on androgen bioactivity in vitro. Molecular & Cellular Endocrinology, 2016;**437**(C):280. doi:10.1016/j.mce.2016.08.041

[45] Cara JF, Rosenfield RL. Insulin-like growth factor I and insulin potentiate luteinizing hormone-induced androgen synthesis by rat ovarian thecal-interstitial cells. Endocrinology. 1988;**123**:733. doi:10.1210/endo-123-2-733

[46] Murray AA, Gosden RG, Allison V, Spears N. Effect of androgens on the development of mouse follicles growing. Journal of Reproduction & Fertility. 1998;**113**:27-33. doi:10.1530/jrf.0.1130027

[47] Pessin JE, Saltiel AR. Signaling pathways in insulin action: molecular targets of insulin resistance. Journal of Clinical Investigation. 2000;**106**:165-169. doi:10.1172/JCI10582

[48] Cheatham B, Kahn CR. Insulin action and the insulin signaling network. Endocrine Reviews. 1995;**16**:117-142. doi:10.1210/er.16.2.117

[49] Kim B, Feldman EL. Insulin resistance as a key link for the increased risk of cognitive impairment in the metabolic syndrome. Experimental & Molecular Medicine. 2015;**47**(3):e149. doi:10.1038/emm.2015.3

[50] Book CB, Dunaif A. Insulin Resistance in the Polycystic Ovary Syndrome[M]//Polycystic Ovary Syndrome. Springer New York. 1996;117-125.

[51] Ciaraldi TP. Molecular mechanisms of insulin resistance in the polycystic ovary syndrome. Contemporary Endocrinology, 2006;**12**:15-20.

[52] Dunaif A. Insulin resistance in women with polycystic ovary syndrome. Fertility & Sterility. 2006;**86**:S13-4. doi:10.1016/j.fertnstert.2006.04.011

[53] Xiao KW, Shan YZ, Jin XL, Pasi P, Kirsimarja S, Marjaana M, Risto E. Selective ovary resistance to insulin signaling in women with polycystic ovary syndrome. Fertility & Sterility. 2003;**80**:954-65. doi:10.1016/S0015-0282(03)01007-0

[54] Xiao KW, Risto E. Ovarian insulin resistance and insulin sensitizer effect on polycystic ovary syndrome. Zhonghua Fu Chan Ke Za Zhi. 2005;**39**:804-808. doi:10.3760/j.issn:0529-567x.2004.12.004

[55] Valavanis IK, Mougiakakou SG, Grimaldi KA, Nikita KS. A multifactorial analysis of obesity as CVD risk factor: Use of neural network based methods in a nutrigenetics context. BMC Bioinformatics. 2010;**11**:453. doi:10.1186/1471-2105-11-453

[56] Pasquali R, Gambineri A, Pagotto U. Review article: The impact of obesity on reproduction in women with polycystic ovary syndrome. Bjog: An International Journal of Obstetrics & Gynaecology. 2006;**113**:1148-1159. doi:10.1111/j.1471-0528.2006.00990.x

[57] Lubrano C, Gnessi L, Migliaccio S. Ovarian function and obesity: PCOS, menopause. Annals of the Rheumatic Diseases. 2015;**63**:386-394. doi:10.1007/978-3-319-09045-0_7

[58] Glueck CJ, Morrison JA, Daniels S, Wang P, Stroop D. Sex hormone-binding globulin, oligomenorrhea, polycystic ovary syndrome, and childhood insulin at age 14 years predict metabolic syndrome and class III obesity at age 24 years. Journal of Pediatrics. 2011;**159**:308-313. doi:10.1016/j.jpeds.2011.01.018

[59] Carmina E, Bucchieri S, Esposito A, Del Puente A, Mansueto P, Orio F, Di Fede G, Rini G. Abdominal fat quantity and distribution in women with polycystic ovary syndrome and extent of its relation to insulin resistance. J Clin Endocrinol Metab. 2007;**92**:2500-2505. doi:10.1210/jc.2006-2725

[60] Baptiste CG, Battista MC, Trottier A, Baillargeon JP. Insulin and hyperandrogenism in women with polycystic ovary syndrome. Journal of Steroid Biochemistry & Molecular Biology. 2010;**122**:42-52. doi:10.1016/j.jsbmb.2009.12.010

[61] Ezeh U, Pall M, Mathur R, Berman D, Chen IY, Dumesic DA, Azziz R. Effects of endogenous androgens and abdominal fat distribution on the interrelationship between insulin and non-insulin-mediated glucose uptake in females. 2013;**98**:1541-8. doi:10.1210/jc.2012-2937

[62] Nascimento JX PT, Chein MBDC, Sousa RMLD, Ferreira ADS, Navarro PA, Brito LMO. Importance of lipid accumulation product index as a marker of CVD risk in PCOS women. Lipids in Health & Disease. 2015;**14**:1-8. doi:10.1186/s12944-015-0061-y

[63] Agarwal A, Aponte-Mellado A, Premkumar BJ, Shaman A, Gupta S. The effects of oxidative stress on female reproduction: A review. Reproductive Biology and Endocrinology. 2012;**10**:1-31. doi:10.1186/1477-7827-10-49

[64] Huang B, Li Z, Ai J, Zhu L, Li Y, Jin L, Zhang H. Antioxidant capacity of follicular fluid from patients undergoing in vitro fertilization. International Journal of Clinical & Experimental Pathology. 2014;**7**:2273-82.

[65] Yilmaz N, Inal HA, Gorkem U, Sargin Oruc A, Yilmaz S, Turkkani A. Follicular fluid total antioxidant capacity levels in PCOS. Journal of Obstetrics & Gynaecology. 2016;**36**(5):1. doi:10.3109/01443615.2016.1148683

[66] Pandey V, Singh A, Singh A, Krishna A, Pandey U, Tripathi YB. Role of oxidative stress and low-grade inflammation in letrozole-induced polycystic ovary syndrome in the rat. Reproductive Biology. 2016;**16**:70. doi:10.1016/j.repbio.2015.12.005

[67] Kaya C, Erkan AF, Cengiz SD, Dünder I, Özlem Erbaş Demirel, Bilgihan A. Advanced oxidation protein products are increased in women with polycystic ovary syndrome: relationship with traditional and nontraditional cardiovascular risk factors in patients with polycystic ovary syndrome. Fertility & Sterility. 2008;**90**(4):1372-7. doi:10.1016/j.fertnstert.2008.08.016

[68] Lin Y, Berg AH, Iyengar P, Lam TK, Giacca A, Combs TP, Rajala MW, Du X, Rollman B, Li W, Hawkins M, Barzilai N, Rhodes CJ, Fantus IG, Brownlee M, Scherer PE. The hyperglycemia-induced inflammatory response in adipocytes: The role of reactive oxygen species. Journal of Biological Chemistry, 2005;**280**(6):4617-26. doi:10.1074/jbc.M411863200

[69] González F, Rote NS, Minium J, Kirwan JP. Reactive oxygen species-induced oxidative stress in the development of insulin resistance and hyperandrogenism in polycystic ovary syndrome. The Journal of Clinical Endocrinology and Metabolism. 2006;**91**:336-40. doi:10.1210/jc.2005-1696

[70] Genxia L, Weiwei L. Relationship between insulin resistance and oxidative stress in patients with PCOS. Journal of Zhengzhou University, 2011;**46**:759-762.doi:10.135/j.issn.1671-6825.2011.05.032

[71] Pourteymour F, Alipoor B, Sadagiani MM, Ostadrahimi A. Effect of Zinc supplementation on cardiometabolic risk factors in women with polycystic ovary syndrome. J Cardiovasc Thorac Res. 2010;**2**:11-20.

[72] Demaria S, Pikarsky E, Karin M, Coussens LM, Yen-Ching C, El-Omar EM, Trinchieri G, Dubinett SM, Mao JT, Szabo E, Krieg A, Weiner GJ, Fox BA, Coukos G, E Wang, Abraham RT, Carbone M, Lotze MT. Cancer and inflammation: promise for biological therapy. Journal of Immunotherapy. 2010;**33**:335-351. doi:10.1097/CJI.0b013e3181d32e74

[73] Paterakis T, Kandarakis HA. Indices of low-grade inflammation in polycystic ovary syndrome. Annals of the New York Academy of Sciences. 2006;**1092**:175-186. doi:10.1196/annals.1365.015

[74] Kelly CC, Lyall H, Petrie JR, Gould GW, Connell JM, Sattar N. Low grade chronic inflammation in women with polycystic ovarian syndrome. Journal of Clinical Endocrinology & Metabolism. 2001;**86**:2453-5. doi:10.1210/jcem.86.6.7580

[75] Ojeda-Ojeda M, Murri M, Insenser M, Escobar-Morreale HF. Mediators of low-grade chronic inflammation in polycystic ovary syndrome (PCOS). Current Pharmaceutical Design. 2013;**19**:5775-91. doi:10.2174/1381612811319320012

[76] Knebel B, Janssen OE, Hahn S, Jacob S, Gleich J, Kotzka J, Muller-Wieland D. Increased low grade inflammatory serum markers in patients with polycystic ovary syndrome (PCOS) and their relationship to PPARgamma gene variants. Experimental & Clinical Endocrinology & Diabetes. 2008;**116**:481-486. doi:10.1055/s-2008-1058085

[77] Nikbakht R, Moramezi F, Farhadi S, Bahman C. Vitamin D deficiency in infertile women with polycystic ovary syndrome: A case–control study. International Journal of Pharmaceutical Research & Allied Science. 2016;**5**:144-150.

[78] Bachali S, Dasu K, Ramalingam K, Naidu JN. Vitamin D deficiency and insulin resistance in normal and type 2 diabetes subjects. Indian Journal of Clinical Biochemistry, 2013;**28**(1):74. doi:10.1007/s12291-012-0239-2

[79] Esteghamati A, Aryan Z, Esteghamati A, Nakhjavani M. Vitamin D deficiency is associated with insulin resistance in nondiabetics and reduced insulin production in type 2 diabetics. Hormone & Metabolic Research. 2014;**47**:273-9. doi:10.1055/s-0034-1389903

[80] Ardabili HR, Gargari BP, Farzadi L. Vitamin D supplementation has no effect on insulin resistance assessment in women with polycystic ovary syndrome and vitamin D deficiency. Nutrition Research. 2012;**32**:195-201. doi:10.1016/j.nutres.2012.02.001

[81] Muscogiuri G, Policola C, Prioletta A, Sorice G, Mezza T, Lassandro A, Della Casa S, Pontecorvi A, Giaccari A. Low levels of 25(OH)D and insulin-resistance: 2 unrelated features or a cause-effect in PCOS? Clinical Nutrition. 2012;**31**:476-480. doi:10.1016/j.clnu.2011.12.010

[82] Holick M F. Vitamin D: important for prevention of osteoporosis, cardiovascular heart disease, type 1 diabetes, autoimmune diseases, and some cancers. South Medical Journal. 2005;**98**:1024-1027. doi: 10.1097/01.SMJ.0000140865.32054.DB

[83] Liu Y, Chen L, Zhi C, Ming S, Weiwei S, Dengshun M, Xiaoqin Y. 1,25(OH)2D3 deficiency induces colon inflammation via secretion of senescence-associated inflammatory cytokines. PLoS One. 2016;**11**(1):e0146426. doi:10.1371/journal.pone.0146426

[84] Wambach CM, Pall ME, Valenton K, Pisarska M, Alexander C. 25-Hydroxy vitamin D3 [25(OH) D] levels are related to BMI in women with polycystic ovary syndrome (PCOS). Fertility & Sterility. 2010;**94**:S199–S199. doi:10.1016/j.fertnstert.2010.07.772

[85] Ujvari D, Hulchiy M, Calaby A, Nybacka Å, Byström B, Hirschberg AL. Lifestyle intervention up-regulates gene and protein levels of molecules involved in insulin signaling in the endometrium of overweight/obese women with polycystic ovary syndrome. Human Reproduction. 2014;**29**:1526-35. doi:10.1093/humrep/deu114

[86] Genazzani A, Battaglia C, Malavasi B, Strucchi C, Tortolani F, Gamba O. Metformin administration modulates and restores luteinizing hormone spontaneous episodic secretion and ovarian function in nonobese patients with polycystic ovary syndrome. Fertility & Sterility. 2004;**81**(1):114-9. doi:10.1016/j.fertnstert.2003.05.020

[87] Dunaif A. Drug insight: Insulin-sensitizing drugs in the treatment of polycystic ovary syndrome—a reappraisal. Nature Clinical Practice Endocrinology & Metabolism, 2008;**4**(5):272-83. doi:10.1038/ncpendmet0787

Chapter 4

Metabolic Disorders Associated with Biological Insulin Resistance in Congolese Woman with Polycystic Ovary Syndrome (PCOS)

Chantal Amisi Anifa, Mputu Lobota,
Mboloko Esimo and Paolo Pozzilli

Additional information is available at the end of the chapter

http://dx.doi.org/10.5772/intechopen.69182

Abstract

We aimed to identify metabolic disorders associated with insulin resistance (IR) in Congolese women affected by polycystic ovary syndrome (PCOS). Fifty-four PCOS women and 40 controls from three hospitals of Kinshasa were enrolled to our case-control study. Blood samples were collected, and concentrations of high-density lipoprotein (HDL) and low-density lipoprotein (LDL) cholesterol, triglycerides (TG), fasting insulin, and glucose levels were measured. IR under basal conditions was evaluated with homeostasis model assessment (HOMA-IR). Dyslipidemia was observed in 37.5 controls and 55.6% PCOS women ($p < 0.05$). The two main lipoproteins concerned were HDL and LDL; nevertheless, the difference in LDL levels between PCOS and controls was not significant. Higher TG (>150 mg/dl) was not found in the two groups, whereas TG levels in PCOS patients were significantly higher than in controls ($p < 0.05$). Impaired glucose tolerance (IGT) and metabolic syndrome were observed, respectively, in 1.9% of PCOS patients. Insulin resistance is associated with metabolic disorders in Congolese woman with PCOS. Dyslipidemia (55.6%), mainly due to low HDL levels, is the most common metabolic disorder. Impaired glucose tolerance and metabolic syndrome represent a small proportion.

Keywords: PCOS, dyslipidemia, insulin resistance, Congolese women, HOMA-IR

1. Introduction

Polycystic ovary syndrome (PCOS) characterized by androgen excess with or without clinical evidence of hyperandrogenism is one of the most common endocrine dysfunctions that affects 5–10% of women of reproductive age [1, 2]. Literature data revealed that PCOS is associated with several metabolic complications, including insulin resistance (IR) with compensatory hyperinsulinemia, impaired glucose tolerance, dyslipidemia, and metabolic syndrome (MS) [2–4].

PCOS women with dyslipidemia show lower HDL and higher TG, without change in LDL [5, 6].

Apridonidze et al. [7] observed that 68% of women had low HDL and 35% higher triglycerides. Another American multicentric study showed lower HDL in 66% of cases and higher TG in 32% of cases [8].

Metabolic syndrome is found in the third part of PCOS women [6, 8–11]. It appears in women with obesity or overweight, suggesting a "knock effect" of the gain of weight, probably in genetically predetermined women [5]. It has been found, respectively, in 43% of PCOS women by Apridonidze et al. [7] and 33.4% by Ehrmann et al. [8].

Likewise, race and age affect the prevalence of IR and metabolic disorders. Therefore, measures used to estimate these features in PCOS patients might take into account these factors.

Currently, few data are available on the prevalence and metabolic disorders of PCOS in African women. Therefore, the present study aimed to determine the frequency and metabolic features associated with IR in Congolese women affected by PCOS using a case-control study.

2. Patients and methods

The present study was carried out from February 2006 to February 2007 in three hospitals of Kinshasa. Fifty-four women with PCOS were recruited while a group of 40 healthy, age matched female subjects were used as controls. Women were all black, African, and from a Congolese ethnic group. Presence of PCOS was defined according to the Rotterdam 2003 consensus [1] by the presence of at least two of the following three features: (1) clinical and/or biochemical signs of hyperandrogenism; (2) oligomenorrhea, that is, menstrual cycles > 45 days or less eight cycles/year and/or anovulation; and (3) presence of polycystic ovaries. Clinical hyperandrogenism was defined by the Ferriman-Gallwey score (F-G score) as > 8. None of these PCOS patients had used hormonal preparation for at least 2 months preceding the study. Control women came from the same ethnic group; they were non-hirsute, without personal or family history of hirsutism and/or endocrine disorders, and free of any treatment. They had regular menstrual cycles, and none of them satisfied any of the PCOS criteria of the Rotterdam 2003 consensus.

PCOS and controls were excluded if they were prepubertal, premenopausal, or pregnant.

All women were subjected to a physical examination including evaluation of blood pressure, weight, abdominal, and hip circumference. Parametric measures included evaluation of body mass index (BMI) and waist-to-hip ratio (WHR). The waist circumference (WC) was defined as the smallest measurement between the iliac crest and lateral costal margin and the hip circumference, as the largest measurement over the buttocks. BMI was defined as body weight in kilograms divided by body height in meters squared (kg/m^2). Overweight was defined as BMI ≥ 25 kg/m^2, and obesity was defined as BMI ≥ 30 kg/m^2, while WHR > 0.85 indicated visceral type of obesity.

2.1. Biochemistry

Capillary glucose was measured using a glucometer (Glucocard, Menarini, Italy). Serum insulin was performed by ELISA using the Mercodia Insulin Elisa kit. We also measured in serum HDL and LDL cholesterol and triglycerides by colometric enzymatic method.

Dyslipidemia was defined by one or more abnormal lipidic fractions using as normal values for LDL ≤ 160, HDL ≥ 50, and triglycerides < 150 mg/dl.

Impaired glucose tolerance (IGT) was defined as fasting hyperglycemia between 110 and 126 mg/dl.

Metabolic syndrome was defined according to Rotterdam 2003 consensus [1] by at least three of the following criteria:

- Abdominal circumference > 88 cm
- Triglycerides ≥ 150 mg/dl
- HDL cholesterol < 50 mg/dl
- Blood pressure ≥ 130/≥ 85 mmHg
- Fasting glucose > 110–126 and/or 2-h of glucose > 140–199 mg/dl

2.2. Statistical analysis

Data were analyzed with commercial software (SPSS version 13.0 for Windows). The Chi-square test, Fisher's exact test, and *t*-test were used to make comparison of quantitative variables and qualitative variables between study groups and sub-groups, according to each case. A p value < 0.05 was considered statistically significant.

3. Results

Table 1 shows the clinical features of PCOS patients and controls. The mean age and BMI were similar in both groups. There was a significant difference for menarche age between the two groups ($p < 0.05$) as well as for the Ferriman & Gallwey (F-G) score ($p < 0.001$), HDL, and TG ($p < 0.05$).

As shown in **Table 2**, dyslipidemia was found among 37.5% of controls and 55.6% of PCOS patients. HDL and LDL were the two lipidic fractions concerned. Lower HDL was the main abnormality observed ($p < 0.001$).

Higher TG (≥ 150 mg/dl) was not found although there was a significant difference between PCOS group and controls (**Table 1**).

Parameters	PCOS (n = 54)	Controls (n = 40)	P
Age	24.54 ± 5.2	23.98 ± 6.3	NS
Menarche age	13.77 ± 1.6	12.62 ± 1.6	<0.05
Ferriman-Gallwey Score	9.46 ± 6.1	3.38 ± 2.4	<0.001
Systolic blood pressure (mmHg)	110.57 ± 13.36	107.25 ± 9.3	NS
Diastolic blood pressure (mmHg)	71.70 ± 12.36	70.50 ± 9.0	NS
BMI	22.0 ± 4.39	22.0 ± 3.32	NS
WC (cm)	76.85 ± 10.9	75.82 ± 8.3	NS
WHR	0.80 ± 0.06	0.77 ± 0.05	NS
Glucose (mg/dl)	78.83 ± 12.7	76.42 ± 10.5	NS
Insulin (μU/L)	13.06 ± 9.1	5.83 ± 3.6	<0.001
HOMA-IR (mol × μU/l^2)	2.62 ± 2.1	1.08 ± 0.67	<0.001
HDL-cholesterol (mg/dl)	49.07 ± 13.72	57.65 ± 16.55	<0.05
LDL-cholesterol (mg/dl)	106.8 ± 31.6	111.10 ± 24.5	NS
Triglycerides (mg/dl)	57.12 ± 21.6	48.52 ± 12.87	<0.05

Table 1. Clinical and biochemical features of the study subjects.

Parameters	PCOS (n = 54)	Controls (n = 40)
HDL-c (mg/dl)		
<50	27 (50%)	14 (35%)
≥50	27 (50%)	25 (65%)
LDL-c (mg/dl)		
<160	49 (90.7%)	39 (97.5%)
≥160	5 (9.3%)	1 (2.5%)
TG (mg/dl)		
<150	54 (100%)	40 (100%)
≥150	0 (0%)	0 (0%)
Dyslipidemia		
Present	30 (55.6%)	15 (37.5%)
Absent	24 (44.4%)	25 (62.5%)

Table 2. Prevalence of dyslipidemia.

Among PCOS women, dyslipidemia varied significantly by waist-to-hip ratio, HDL, and TG.

PCOS patients identified as having dyslipidemia were compared with those without dyslipidemia. Overall, PCOS patients with dyslipidemia had the same age and LDL level but lower HDL and higher TG level. In addition, they had greater android body fat distribution. There was no difference in the HOMA-IR index, although patients with dyslipidemia showed higher level of this parameter (**Table 3**).

Impaired glucose tolerance as well as metabolic syndrome was observed in only one PCOS women.

Parameters	PCOS with dyslipidemia (n = 30)	PCOS without dyslipidemia (n = 24)	P
WHR	0.81 ± 0.05	0.78 ± 0.06	<0.05
HDL-c	40.70 ± 10.09	59.53 ± 9.98	<0.001
LDL-c	111.63 ± 34.5	100.76 ± 27.2	NS
TG	63.6 ± 23.4	49.02 ± 16.1	<0.05
HOMA-IR	2.8 ± 2.3	2.4 ± 1.7	NS

Table 3. Variations of dyslipidemia among PCOS subjects.

4. Discussion

In our knowledge, this is the first study that describes lipid and lipoprotein profile and metabolic disorders associated to IR in Congolese women with PCOS.

We determined lipids and lipoprotein levels which were in the normal range. Our results are in accordance with previous African studies which had found lower levels of lipid and lipoprotein in African people compared to values reported in Caucasians [12–16, 22]. This difference could be explained by the low-fat and high-carbohydrate African diet. Indeed, nutritional transition is in process in Kinshasa. Although few people have modified their diet, eating more and more refined sugar and animal fat and less vegetable, the diet in people from Kinshasa remains poor in fat and wealthy in carbohydrates.

We observed in our study among PCOS women lower HDL and higher TG without change in LDL and this is consistent with other previous reports [7, 8, 17]. This inverse relation between HDL and TG is commonly found in insulin resistance and hyperinsulinemia.

We failed to observe a significant association between metabolic syndrome and biological insulin resistance as reported by several authors [5, 7, 8, 18, 19], possibly owing to the TG level ≥ 150 mg/dl in the metabolic syndrome's definition that we used. In addition, the small number of obeses in our PCOS group could also explain this observation. Previous studies have reported greater proportion of obesity and overweight subjects. Indeed, the prevalence of metabolic syndrome increases with the rise of BMI [9, 10, 18, 20]. Overall, 30–50% of obesity or overweight can be found in women with PCOS. In the USA, more than 30% of adults are obese [5, 21]. In our study, only 3.7% of PCOS women were obese.

We observed the so-called TG paradox that has been described in Sub-Saharan African populations: normal triglycerides levels in the presence of IR [22].

The generally accepted cut-off point of TG level (≥ 150 mg/dl) could underestimate dyslipidemia and metabolic syndrome in African people due to lower lipid and lipoprotein levels reported in several African studies [12–16, 22]. It is, therefore, important to describe African lipid and lipoprotein profile and to propose another definition of metabolic syndrome, either in PCOS and in other patients. These findings may allow to discover existing metabolic syndrome in most of the PCOS patients from our study that could not be determined using international lipid and lipoprotein levels and the Rotterdam 2003 metabolic syndrome definition.

There were inherent limitations associated with this study: one of them was the limited number of patients. However, given the paucity of data available on PCOS in African women, our data, even though collected among a limited number of patients, confirm the need for further knowledge in endocrine and metabolic diseases in developing countries.

5. Conclusion

It is concluded that insulin resistance is associated with metabolic disorders in Congolese woman with PCOS. Dyslipidemia (55.6%), mainly due to low HDL levels, is the most common metabolic disorder. Impaired glucose tolerance and metabolic syndrome represent a small proportion.

Author details

Chantal Amisi Anifa[1]*, Mputu Lobota[2], Mboloko Esimo[2] and Paolo Pozzilli[1]

*Address all correspondence to: chantalamisi@yahoo.fr

1 Università Campus Bio-Medico di Roma, Rome, Italy

2 University Clinics of Kinshasa, Kinshasa, The Democratic Republic of Congo

References

[1] The Rotterdam ESHRE/ASRM sponsored PCOS consensus workshop group. Revised 2003 consensus on diagnostic criteria and long-term health risks related to polycystic ovary syndrome. Hum Reprod 2004;**19**:41-47

[2] Alexander CJ, Tangchitnob EP, Lepor NE. Polycystic ovary syndrome: A major unrecognized cardiovascular risk factor in women. Reviews in Obstetrics & Gynecology. 2009;**2**(4):232-239

[3] Dunaif A, Segal KR, Futterweit W, Dobransky A. Profound peripheral insulin resistance, independent of obesity, in polycystic ovary syndrome. Diabetes. 1989;**38**:1165-1174

[4] Lobo RA, Carmina E. The importance of diagnosing the polycystic ovary syndrome. Annals of Internal Medicine. 2000;**132**:989-993

[5] Moraillon M, Gompel A. Syndrome des ovaires micropolykystiques et risque cardiovasculaire. Sang Thrombose Vaisseaux. 2007;**19**:65-75

[6] Rocha MP, et al. Dyslipidemia in women with polycystic ovary syndrome: Incidence, pattern and predictors. Gynecological Endocrinology. 2011;**27**(10):814-819

[7] Apridonidze T, Essah PA, Iuorno MJ, Nestler JE. Prevalence and characteristics of the metabolic syndrome in women with polycystic ovary syndrome. Journal of Clinical Endocrinology & Metabolism. 2005;**90**:1929-1935

[8] Ehrmann DA, Liljenquist DR, Kasza K, Azziz R, Legro RS, Ghazzi MN, PCOS/Troglitazone Study Group. Prevalence and predictors of the metabolic syndrome in women with polycystic ovary syndrome. Journal of Clinical Endocrinology & Metabolism. 2006;**91**:48-53

[9] Coney P, Ladson G, Sweet S, Legro RS. Does polycystic ovary syndrome increase the disparity in metabolic syndrome and cardiovascular-related health for African-American women? Seminars in Reproductive Medicine. 2008;**26**(1):35-38

[10] Coviello AD, Legro RS, Dunaif A. Adolescent girls with polycystic ovary syndrome have an increased risk of the metabolic syndrome associated with increasing androgen levels independent of obesity and insulin resistance. Journal of Clinical Endocrinology & Metabolism. 2006;**91**:492-497

[11] Weerakiet S, et al. Prevalence of the metabolic syndrome in Asian women with polycystic ovary syndrome: Using the International Diabetes Federation criteria. Gynecological Endocrinology. 2007;**23**(3):153-160

[12] Lepira FB, Mbuyamba-Kabangu JR, Kayembe KP, Nseka MN. Correlates of serum lipids and lipoproteins in Congolese patients with arterial hypertension. Cardiovascular Journal of Africa. 2005;**16**:249-255

[13] Fasanmade O, Oke D, Odeniyi I, Okafor C. Pattern of dyslipidemia amongst Nigerians with type 2 diabetes mellitus. Diabetic Medicine. 2006;**23**(Suppl. 4):110-111

[14] Ehusani-Anumah F, Fasanmade O, Bello-Sani F, Danbauchi S, Oyati I, Alhassan M, Adeyemi-Doro A. Influence of type 2 diabetes on the profiles of Northern Nigerians. Diabetic Medicine. 2006;**23**(Suppl. 4):110

[15] Coker A, Adeyemi-Doro O, Fasanmade O, Ezeani N, Ohwovoriole A. Determinants of dyslipidaemia in a selection of Nigerians with type 2 diabetes mellitus. Diabetic Medicine. 2006;**23**(Suppl. 4):109

[16] Akwo E, Nwatsock J, Ashuntantang G, Ndip A, Effoe V, Sobngwi E, Mbanya J. Prevalence and clinical significance of dyslipidaemia in a population of Sub-Saharan type 2 diabetic patients. Diabetic Medicine. 2006;**23**(Suppl. 4):109

[17] Strowitzki T, Halser B, Demant T. Body fat distribution, insulin sensitivity, ovarian dysfunction and serum lipoproteins in patients with polycystic ovary syndrome. Gynecological Endocrinology. 2002;**16**:45-51

[18] Buysschaert M. Le syndrome métabolique: Nouvelles définitions et conséquences. Louvain Médical. 2006;**125**:79-81

[19] Colin IM. Obésité, Syndrome métabolique et Diabète: Les complices désignés d'une épidémie d'un genre nouveau. Louvain Médical. 2005;**124**:7-10

[20] Alberti KGMM, Zimmet P, Shaw J. For the IDF epidemiology task force consensus group: The metabolic syndrome—a new worldwide definition. Lancet. 2005;**366**:1059-1062

[21] Bhattacharya SM. Prevalence of metabolic syndrome in women with polycystic ovary syndrome, using two proposed definitions. Gynecological Endocrinology. 2010;**26**(7):516-520

[22] Yu SS, Castillo DC, Courville AB, Sumner AE. The triglyceride paradox in people of African descent. Metabolic Syndrome and Related Disorders. 2012;**10**(2):77-82

Chapter 5

Fertility Treatment for Women with PCOS

Fiona Langdon, Jennifer Pontre and Roger J. Hart

Additional information is available at the end of the chapter

http://dx.doi.org/10.5772/intechopen.71188

Abstract

Polycystic ovarian syndrome is the commonest cause of anovulatory infertility. This chapter will explore fertility treatment options for this condition including the risks, benefits and success rates for different treatment methods. The importance of close patient monitoring with hormone levels and pelvic ultrasounds to ensure mono-ovulation and to avoid ovarian hyperstimulation syndrome will be highlighted.

Keywords: polycystic ovary syndrome, anovulation, obesity, ovulation induction, ovarian hyperstimulation, gonadotrophins

1. Introduction

Polycystic ovarian syndrome (PCOS) is the commonest cause of anovulatory infertility [1]. Depending on the population studied between 5 and 18% of women of reproductive age suffer from PCOS, however not all of them are anovulatory or experience subfertility [2–4].

The aim of fertility treatment in women with subfertility and PCOS is to safely induce mono-follicular ovulation resulting in the birth of a singleton child. Women undergoing fertility treatment with PCOS are at significant risk of both multi-follicular development and ovarian hyper-stimulation syndrome (OHSS), so they must be carefully counselled and monitored during fertility treatment. It is imperative that prior to embarking on fertility treatment a patient's health and weight is optimised. This chapter will explore the latest evidence for fertility treatments for women with PCOS.

2. Definition and diagnosis of PCOS

The current diagnosis for PCOS surrounds the cluster of signs and symptoms that the syndrome encompasses, namely anovulation, hyperandrogenaemia, insulin resistance and polycystic ovaries. The Rotterdam Criteria for diagnosis of PCOS requires two of the three diagnostic criteria, namely oligo- or anovulation, clinical or biochemical signs of hyperandrogenism and polycystic ovarian morphology (**Table 1**) [1].

There is discussion that the Rotterdam criteria is too broad and may be resulting in over diagnosis of the syndrome [5], especially in young women, prone to clinical signs of hyperandrogenism and who are more likely to have morphological features of polycystic ovaries on USS. Furthermore, when investigating a patient for possible PCOS, age, ethnicity and weight should be factored in.

Hyperandrogenic features, either biochemical or chemical, are seen in 60–80% of patients with PCOS [6]. Clinical features of hyperandrogenism correlate poorly with blood androgen levels, especially in some ethnic groups, particularly South East Asian, with increased sebaceous gland susceptibility to circulating androgens. Serum androgen concentrations must be measured in the setting of more severe clinical findings to ensure other causes of hirsutism are excluded such as adrenal tumours or non-classical congenital adrenal hyperplasia (CAH).

Polycystic ovarian morphology definition is predominantly based on findings from a paper by Sonnard in 2003 comparing 214 ovaries of PCOS patients with 112 normal women's ovaries to conclude that a diagnosis of polycystic ovaries should be more than 12 follicles measuring between 2 and 9 mm per ovary or an ovarian volume of more than $10cm^3$. This diagnostic criterion is now largely seen to be too broad with further studies and improvement in ultrasound techniques suggesting that either the diagnostic follicle number should be increased [7] or raised AMH levels should be included in the diagnostic criteria.

Oligo-ovulation or anovulation is suggested by either irregular cycles or a sup-optimal mid-luteal phase progesterone. Cycles that are either shorter than 21 days or longer than 35 days are highly suggestive of anovulation, although It is recognised that even in adolescents with very short or protracted cycles ovulation can still occur, with obvious implications should pregnancy avoidance be required [8].

Two out of the following three criteria
1. Oligo- and/or anovulation
2. Clinical and/or biochemical signs of hyperandrogenism
3. Polycystic ovaries on ultrasound after exclusion of other aetiologies (congenital adrenal hyperplasia, androgen secreting tumours, Cushing's syndrome)

Table 1. Revised ESHRE/ASRM Rotterdam consensus diagnostic criteria for PCOS.

3. Lifestyle modifications and weight loss

The first line of treatment and advice to women with PCOS seeking fertility treatment should be to optimise health. This is true for all women considering pregnancy but imperative for women with PCOS due to the commonly seen associations of obesity and metabolic disorders. Furthermore, as with any woman about to start to try to conceive, her doctor must stabilise any co-existing morbidities, and any medication prescribed must be safe for pregnancy.

While 9–18% of the female reproductive age population meet the criteria for PCOS, up to 70% of obese women do [9]. Obese patients with PCOS have an associated increase in severity of the disease, not just from a fertility perspective but for all metabolic and psychological sequelae of the disorder, when compared with non-obese PCOS patients. Obesity is associated with an increased risk of anovulation, increased androgen production and decreased response to follicular stimulating hormone (FSH) equating to decreased fecundity both in natural conception and assisted reproductive techniques [10]. Risks to the foetus if conception does occur include increased rates of congenital anomalies (neural tube defects, omphalocele and cardiac defects) [11], increased rates of hypoglycaemia of the newborn and other complications of gestational diabetes and long-term greater risks of metabolic disease for life. Risks to the pregnant obese patient include greater incidence of hypertensive disorders in pregnancy, increased incidence of thromboembolic events, increased incidence of gestational diabetes, increased risks of operative delivery and increased risks of perineal trauma [11]. For all these reasons, it is imperative that patients embarking on fertility treatment are first counselled and advised to optimise their weight and aim for a body mass index (BMI) in the healthy range.

With a 5–10% weight reduction in patients with PCOS significant benefits are seen in all aspects of health, including reproductive health. Spontaneous ovulation is more likely and patient's response to fertility treatment is more likely to be successful [12, 13]. Caloric restriction, increased physical activity and weight loss medication can all play a role in helping patients achieve the necessary weight loss to either conceive spontaneously or have greater success with fertility treatments. There is limited data on live birth rates, however a loss of weight from an unhealthy weight range in PCOS patients is associated with an improved waist to hip ratio measurement, improved clinical and biochemical signs of hyperandrogenism and improved insulin resistance [14].

A recent randomised control trial of 149 patients with PCOS and body mass index (BMI) between 27 and 41 kg/m^2 compared 16 weeks of lifestyle modification (caloric restriction, weight loss medication and increased levels of physical activity), the combined oral contraceptive pill (COCP) or both interventions followed by 4 cycles of clomiphene citrate and timed intercourse. The researchers found significant weight loss in the lifestyle modification group (mean weight loss −6.2%) and the combined group (mean weight loss −6.4%) when compared to the COCP only group. Superior cumulative ovulation rates were seen in the lifestyle group (60%) and the combined group (67%) compared with the COCP group (46%) after 4 cycles of clomiphene citrate. Live birth rates were not significantly increased, although the study was not adequately powered for livebirth as an outcome, but were higher in the lifestyle (26%) and combined (24%) group compared with the COCP group (12%) [12].

Bariatric surgery can be considered in women with a BMI over 35 and who have had a failed attempt at weight loss with lifestyle modifications. Bariatric surgery improves markers of PCOS influencing fertility, namely anovulatory cycles, hormonal ratios and insulin resistance, but comes with the increased risk of a malabsorptive state and disordered eating as well as psychological issues [15–17]. There are limited trials powered to confirm an absolute improvement in live birth rates following bariatric surgery. Pregnancy and fertility treatments should be avoided for a minimum of 12 months after such surgery to reduce the pregnancy complications associated with bariatric surgery, such as; preterm birth and being small for gestational age. This is due to the profound catabolic state existing after surgery and the depletion of micro-nutrients from the diet [18]. Due to this enforced time delay, in the setting of an older woman with falling ovarian reserve, time for substantial weight loss or bariatric surgery may not be feasible to ensure a successful pregnancy. In these cases, with proper counselling, more leniency may be given to cut off levels of BMI to commence fertility treatment.

4. Metformin

Metformin is a biguanide antihyperglycaemic medication used in Type 2 diabetes mellitus. It acts by decreasing glucose levels through reducing hepatic glucose production and reducing intestinal absorption of glucose, overall reducing the level of insulin secretion. As PCOS has a strong association with hyperinsulinaemia and insulin resistance many patients with PCOS have been treated with metformin, and there is a substantial amount of research showing the beneficial effects of metformin on reproductive outcomes. There is strong evidence to show that within 1–3 months of commencing metformin treatment there is improvement in cycle regularity and improved ovulation rates [19]. Up to 50% of anovulatory women with PCOS will ovulate after treatment with metformin [20]. It is thought metformin acts by not only reducing insulin levels systemically, but also by directly acting on the ovary to alter gonadotrophin levels [21]. Metformin use is associated with weight loss, greater than with lifestyle changes alone, and thus is associated with the reproductive benefits outlined in the weight loss effects above [22].

Metformin's influence on reproductive outcomes has demonstrated an improvement in clinical pregnancy rates, without an improvement in overall live birth rates, and does not appear to provide additional benefit when combined with clomiphene citrate, unless used in the profoundly overweight patient. A meta-analysis of 38 trials of nearly 3500 women showed that there was no increase in the live birth rate for women treated with metformin, either as a single agent (OR1.80 CI 0.52–6.16) or as an addition to clomiphene citrate. (OR 1.16, CI 0.85–1.56) [23].

However there is some evidence that metformin may improve live birth rates for women undergoing ovulation induction when combined with gonadotrophins. Two RCTS comparing the use of placebo versus metformin in ovulation induction with gonadotrophins for women with PCOS have shown a higher live birth rate (OR 2.31) in the metformin and gonadotrophin group compared with the placebo and gonadotrophin group, however the numbers studied were small [24, 25]. There was no observed increase in multiple pregnancy rates in these studies or others looking at clinical pregnancy rates only, with the addition of metformin [26].

From the studies outlined above metformin cannot be recommended as a treatment for ovulation induction alone, however in obese or overweight women it can play a role in weight loss which may facilitate spontaneous ovulation in conjunction with clomiphene. There is some limited data that it may improve reproductive outcomes as an adjunct to ovulation induction treatment with gonadotrophins in women with diagnosed PCOS.

5. Clomiphene and anti-oestrogens

Clomiphene citrate is a selective oestrogen receptor modulator (SERM) used to induce ovulation in anovulatory patients for over 50 years [27]. It will induce ovulation in around 75% of patients with PCOS. Increasing doses of clomiphene results in increased rates of ovulation, but not necessarily increased rates of pregnancy. Being a SERM, clomiphene acts on oestrogen receptors in the hypothalamus and pituitary, to increase follicular stimulating hormone (FSH) production, and on receptors in the endometrium and cervix with differing antagonist and agonist qualities depending on dose [28]. Clomiphene, particularly in higher doses, can produce a less receptive endometrial environment and a more hostile cervical mucus, which may negatively affect pregnancy rates.

Ovulation rates were studied at different doses for women with PCOS, with the finding that at a starting dose of 50 mg per day 46% of patients ovulate, 70% ovulate with 100 mg, 76% with 150 mg and up to 90% at doses greater than 150 mg daily for 5 days [29]. As doses increase a lower percentage of the women who have not ovulated previously on the lower dose have success with the higher dose as the proportion of women with true clomiphene resistance increases. Patients are usually deemed clomiphene resistant, thought to affect around 15% of women with PCOS, if no follicle development is seen with 3 cycles of maximal dose (150 mg for 5 days) of clomiphene citrate [30]. Patients are more likely to be clomiphene resistant if they are obese and suffer from significant hyperandrogenism [31].

Evidence suggests women with PCOS undergoing fertility treatment with clomiphene have a cumulative pregnancy rate of around 45% after 4 cycles and 65% after 6 cycles [32], with a live birth rate of around 42% [33]. After 6 cycles of treatment the pregnancy rate falls despite regular ovulation, suggesting other subfertility issues may be present in the couple or the effects of high dose clomiphene is impacting the uterus.

It is essential that clomiphene treatment, as with any ovulation induction treatment, must be monitored with serial transvaginal ultrasound examinations (TVUS) to monitor follicular development, and allow for cycle cancellation if a response with more than one dominant follicle developing is seen. Monitoring treatment in this way keeps the rate of multiple pregnancies to a minimum. The multiple pregnancy rate with clomiphene treatment is between 6.9–9% for twin pregnancies and less than 1% for higher order multiple pregnancy. Congenital malformations have not been shown to be any higher in women taking clomiphene than women who spontaneously ovulated [34].

Clomiphene treatment is for the most part well tolerated with common side effects relating to the effects of hypoestrogenism including hot flushes, abdominal distention, nausea and breast tenderness being seen in 10–20% of patients. Side effects do not appear to be dose dependent, but rather a result of patient response.

The risk of ovarian hyperstimulation syndrome (OHSS) is theoretical with clomiphene use and if occurs is nearly always mild. Treatment dose should always be started low and increased only if ovulation has not occurred to avoid this risk.

Clomiphene has been the first line fertility treatment for women with PCOS for many years, however data is emerging that other treatment modalities have greater success and a move away from using clomiphene citrate in the first instance is being practiced.

6. Letrozole

Letrozole is an aromatase inhibitor inducing a hypo-oestrogen state by inhibiting the enzyme converting androgens to oestrone and oestradiol. A low serum oestradiol concentration results in increased pituitary FSH production, and consequently subsequent follicular development and ovulation. It is licenced for the treatment of oestrogen sensitive breast cancers in postmenopausal women, but is gaining popularity in its currently off label use in producing mono-ovulation in women undergoing fertility treatment with PCOS.

Like clomiphene, letrozole is given in the early follicular phase of the cycle for 5 consecutive days. Dosing is started low, usually at 2.5 mg to ensure response can be monitored and avoid cycle cancellation if an exaggerated follicular response is seen. Higher doses are associated with poorer endometrial thickness, but not at the levels seen with clomiphene citrate [35].

Compared with clomiphene citrate letrozole has been shown in a randomised controlled trial and a meta-analysis of six trials to be superior at inducing ovulation (the RCT showing relative risk (RR)1.28) and live-birth rates (RR 1.44) [36, 37]. These results were particularly evident for patients with a body mass index over 30 kg/m^2, with no significant difference between the two treatment modalities in patients with a BMI of less than 30 kg/m^2. The same study reported lower multiple pregnancy rates with letrozole compared with clomiphene use (3.4% vs. 7.4%), however the study was not powered for this outcome.

http://dx.doi.org/10.5772/intechopen.71188

Studies looking at foetal safety with letrozole use have found no significant difference in the rates of congenital anomalies in pregnancies conceived using letrozole, compared with clomiphene or spontaneous ovulation [38]. Side effects related to low oestrogen levels with letrozole appear to be less common than those seen with clomiphene use.

Particularly for patients who are obese (BMI over 30 kg/m^2) letrozole can be considered as a first line treatment for mono-ovulation induction. For women with a BMI less than 30 kg/m^2 letrozole may lead to similar pregnancy rates to clomiphene, however the side effect profile and the possible lower multiple pregnancy rates may favour the use of letrozole.

7. Gonadotrophins

Gonadotrophins in the form of injectable recombinant FSH are used in women with PCOS to induce mono-ovulation, historically as a second-line treatment after a patient had failed clomiphene citrate treatment. The perceived risk of ovarian hyper-stimulation and multiple gestation has meant it has been overlooked as a first-line treatment. This view is changing with more evidence to support its use, particularly with low dose, step-up protocols with very close monitoring (Langdon et al. 2017 personal communication).

Patients with PCOS are particularly sensitive to FSH due to the high antral follicle count associated with the condition. It is imperative that the dose threshold to induce ovulation is reached gradually to reduce the risk of multiple follicles being recruited resulting in cycle cancellation, multiple pregnancy or even OHSS, as well as patient disappointment. In therapy naïve patients dosing usually begins at 25 or 37.5 IU/day increasing by small increments (usually 12.5 IUI) at a minimum of 7–10 days, if no response is seen on vaginal ultrasound monitoring or serum oestradiol levels [39]. Requirements for higher doses of FSH are often seen in women with a greater BMI, older age, insulin resistance and amenorrhoea compared with oligomenorrhoea [33].

The success of gonadotrophin ovulation induction is superior to clomiphene. An RCT of therapy naïve women with PCOS compared to treatment with either clomiphene or low dose FSH for up to 3 cycles and found that treatment with FSH had a higher first cycle pregnancy rate (30% vs. 14.6%, 95% CI 5.3–25.8), overall pregnancy rate (58% vs. 44%, 95% CI 1.5–25.8) and live birth rate (47.4% vs. 36.9%.) [42].

Despite the increased success rates associated with gonadotrophin use the therapy has not been embraced as a routine first line fertility treatment for PCOS in many fertility centres due to older studies warning of increased complication rates with its use, and a lack of reimbursement in some jurisdictions. Multiple gestation rates when FSH is used with the purpose of achieving of mono-ovulation are documented to be as low as 6%, comparable to clomiphene use [40]. This is achieved by strictly adhering to a low dose, slow step-up protocol as outlined above. It is further achieved by being wary of patients who may have a greater response to FSH treatment, namely younger patients, those with high AMH levels and those with normal BMI, and ensuring treatment is commenced on the lowest FSH dose possible, and only increased after a period of up to 14 days with no response. Cancelling cycles when response is excessive is imperative to keeping multiple pregnancy rates down. Having a 5–20% cancellation rate has been shown to be associated with a less than 2% higher order multiple pregnancy rate and no difference in pregnancy rates over 4 cycles, and patients should be thoroughly counselled about this [41].

OHSS is a risk with FSH use but with carefully monitored use as described above in women with PCOS the risk is minimal and almost completely avoidable. The risk is only present if too many follicles are stimulated, thus starting with a low dose of FSH, and making small incremental increases only when no response is seen over an extended period and having a low threshold for cancellation of the cycle, OHSS risk can be completely avoided.

A review of 591 cycles of ovulation induction with gonadotrophins in 268 PCOS patients in our unit demonstrated that adherence to a low dose step up protocol had success rates of 22% for their first cycle, 18% for second cycles and 7% for third cycles. Success rates fell steeply after a third cycle. Success rates were highest for women with normal BMI (<25 kg/m^2) and aged less than 35 years. Our multiple pregnancy rate was 2% with a cancellation rate of 13%. Over 591 cycles there were no cases of OHSS (Langdon et al. 2017, personal communication).

With careful administration and monitoring of a low-dose step up protocol, FSH ovulation induction is more successful and not associated with any greater risk than clomiphene. Many units are moving towards using this method as a first line treatment for PCOS patients. It is worth noting that success rates seem to fall after 3 cycles and consideration should be given to attempting other forms of fertility treatment if pregnancy has not been achieved by this point.

8. Laparoscopic ovarian drilling

Laparoscopic ovarian drilling is a longstanding treatment for anovulation for women with PCOS. It is of value if performed at the time of diagnostic laparoscopy as part of a general infertility investigation after fallopian tube patency has been demonstrated and a normal semen assessment has been documented. It also offers rural patients the ability to undergo ovulation induction treatment without the requirement for frequent blood tests and ultrasound examinations. Laparoscopic ovarian drilling improves ovulation rates likely through destruction of theca cells in the ovary that produce androgens resulting in increased FSH levels and reduced LH levels conducive to normal follicular development. As a first line treatment, randomised trials have shown similar results for ovulation, conception and live birth rates when compared with up to 6 cycles of clomiphene [42] and has a likely ongoing success rate without the risk of multiple pregnancy from clomiphene.

Compared with gonadotrophins, similar rates of pregnancy and live birth rate were seen in a meta-analysis of randomised trials comparing the two methods but with far lower multiple pregnancies and no risk of OHSS [43]. Potential drawbacks of laparoscopic ovarian drilling include the possibility of pelvic adhesion development and possible reduction in ovarian reserve. Studies looking at repeat laparoscopies following ovarian drilling procedures have shown adhesions in over 30% of patients treated with diathermy and 50% of patients treated with laser [44]. Reduced serum AMH concentrations, antral follicle counts, and ovarian volume as well as raised FSH levels following ovarian drilling support the notion that ovarian drilling has a possible negative impact on ovarian reserve.

9. In vitro fertilisation (IVF) and reducing OHSS rates

In vitro fertilisation (IVF) is usually reserved for women with PCOS who have failed other treatments or with additional issues compromising their fertility. Women with PCOS, as has been discussed previously, are especially at risk of developing OHSS when undergoing IVF, but as a consequence of this often respond very well to IVF stimulation producing many follicles and oocytes. It is a careful balance to ensure a patient responds well to FSH dosing, but not so well that they are at significant risk of OHSS. A patient with PCOS undergoing an IVF stimulation cycle needs to have a well monitored, individualised stimulation regime to reduce the risk of OHSS and minimise the chance of cycle cancellation. Her age, antral follicle count, anti-Mullerian hormone level (AMH) and BMI should all be considered when starting a cycle and planning the starting dose of FSH. Monitoring with transvaginal ultrasound and serum oestradiol concentrations should be very thorough with a low threshold for cancelling a cycle or employing other methods to reduce the risk of OHSS.

Other ways of avoiding OHSS in these high-risk patients is to routinely use GnRH antagonists rather than agonists to prevent the LH surge [45]. Two meta-analyses have shown lower rates of OHSS when GnRH antagonists are used compared to use of an agonist, but possibly at the cost of slightly reduced pregnancy rates as GnRH agonists generally result in enhanced follicle recruitment [46, 47].

Coasting can be a way to prevent cancellation of the cycle if oestrogen levels are rising too rapidly and there is concern the patient may be at risk of OHSS. Coasting involves withholding FSH therapy while continuing LH suppression with a GnRH agonist or antagonist. This is done until oestradiol levels fall to an acceptable level, if they do not a low threshold must be maintained to cancel the cycle. A review employing 3 days of coasting in the event of high oestradiol levels had minimal effect on pregnancy rates and importantly a low OHSS rate (<2%) [48]. If coasting occurred for longer than 3 days pregnancy rates were affected and thus the suggestion is made that after 3 days of coasting if oestradiol levels have not fallen, consideration of cycle cancellation is warranted.

There is growing evidence of the benefits of metformin use prior to IVF cycles in women with PCOS to reduce the risk of OHSS. Two meta-analyses have found similar results with a significant reduction in OHSS rates in patients pre-treated with metformin (OR 0.27, 95%CI 0.16–0.46 and OR 0.29, 95%CI 0.18–0.49) [49, 50], although metformin treatment was not shown to affect the live birth rate compared with placebo treatment in either study.

Selection of patients	
	IVF only in appropriately selected patients following unsuccessful ovulation induction or other specific fertility issues requiring treatment with IVF
	Consideration of in vitro oocyte maturation in very high risk patients
	Pre-treatment with Metformin and continue through IVF cycle
Cycle management	
	Well monitored, individualised stimulation regime
	Low threshold for cycle cancellation
	GnRH antagonist protocol
	Consider cycle coasting for up to 3 days if concern high for OHSS
At time of trigger injection	
	Use an agonist trigger and adopt a "freeze-all embryos" approach to the cycle
	Consideration of the use of a dopamine agonist to reduce OHSS risk
Luteal phase management	
	Continue ovarian down-regulation into the luteal phase if no embryo transfer is planned
	Early consideration of adopting a "freeze-all" approach
	If proceeding to a fresh embryo transfer: *the replacement of a single embryo*

Table 2. Methods for reduction of rates of OHSS in women with PCOS undergoing IVF.

In vitro oocyte maturation (IVM) is a new technique that eliminates the risk of OHSS [51] and is well suited to patients with PCOS due to their high antral follicle count. Immature oocytes are collected and matured in culture before undergoing either IVF or ICSI fertilisation techniques. It requires minimal amounts of stimulation prior to antral follicle collection eradicating the risk of OHSS and also reducing medication costs to the patient. Data suggests that the live birth rate may be reduced in comparison with standard IVF cycles, especially in fresh cycles, however for frozen embryo transfer cycles pregnancy, miscarriage and live birth rates are not significantly different [52].

It is imperative that clinicians who put women with PCOS through IVF stimulation cycles are vigilant for the development of OHSS in these patients and monitor and treat accordingly (**Table 2**).

10. Conclusion

PCOS is the most common cause of anovulatory infertility and thus is responsible for a large percentage of women seeking fertility treatment. When implementing a treatment plan for a patient with PCOS their metabolic health and weight are important factors that must be

http://dx.doi.org/10.5772/intechopen.71188

addressed and managed prior to embarking on assisted reproductive techniques. The risks of OHSS and multi-follicular development in patients with PCOS means that care must be taken with close, careful monitoring to ensure mono-ovulation is achieved and the risks of multiple pregnancy and OHSS is kept to a minimum. If this approach is adopted the infertility treatment for these women is both safe and effective and patients should be reassured of these facts.

Author details

Fiona Langdon[1,2], Jennifer Pontre[1] and Roger J. Hart[2,3]*

*Address all correspondence to: roger.hart@uwa.edu.au

1 King Edward Memorial Hospital, Perth, WA, Australia

2 Fertility Specialists of Western Australia, Bethesda Hospital, WA, Australia

3 Division of Obstetrics and Gynaecology, University of Western Australia, Women and Infants Research Foundation, King Edward Memorial Hospital, Perth, WA, Australia

References

[1] ESHRE Capri Working Group. Health and fertility in World Health Organization group 2 anovulatory women. Human Reproduction Update. 2012;**18**:586-599

[2] ESHRE REA-SPCWG. Revised 2003 consensus on diagnostic criteria and long term health risks related to polycystic ovary syndrome (PCOS). Human Reproduction. 2004;**19**:41-47

[3] March WA, et al. The prevalence of polycystic ovary syndrome in a community assessed under contrasting diagnostic criteria. Human Reproduction. 2010;**25**:544-551

[4] Hart R, Hickey M, Franks S. Definitions, prevalence and symptoms of polycystic ovaries and polycystic ovary syndrome. Best Practice & Research. Clinical Obstetrics & Gynaecology. 2004 Oct;**18**(5):671-683

[5] Wang R, Mol BWJ. The Rotterdam criteria for polycystic ovary syndrome: Evidence-based criteria? Human Reproduction. 2017;**32**(2):261-264

[6] Balen AH, et al. The management of anovulatory infertility in women with polycystic ovary syndrome: An analysis of the evidence to support the development of global WHO guidance. Human Reproduction Update. 2016;**22**(6):687-708

[7] Dewailly D, et al. Definition and significance of polycystic ovarian morphology: A task force report from the androgen excess and polycystic ovary syndrome society. Human Reproduction Update. 2014;**20**:334-352

[8] PeÃ AAS, Doherty DA, Atkinson HC, Hickey M, Norman RJ, Hart R. The majority of irregular menstrual cycles in adolescence are ovulatory: Results of a prospective study. Archives of Disease in Childhood. 2017. DOI: 10.1136/archdischild-2017-312968 Published Online First: [9th 8 August 2017]

[9] Vrbikova J, et al. Obesity and polycystic ovary syndrome. Obesity Facts. 2009;**2**:26-35

[10] Perales-Puchalt A, Legro RS. Ovulation induction in women with polycystic ovary syndrome. Steroids. 2013;**78**:767-772

[11] Doherty DA, Newnham JP, Bower C, Hart R. Implications of polycystic ovary syndrome for pregnancy and for the health of the offspring. Obstetrics and Gynecology. 2015;**125**(6):1397-1406

[12] Legro RS, et al. Randomised controlled trial of preconception interventions in infertile women with polycystic ovary syndrome. The Journal of Clinical Endocrinology and Metabolism. 2015;**100**:4048-4058

[13] Palomba S, et al. Six weeks of structured exercise training and hypocaloric diet increases the probability of ovulation after clomiphene citrate in overweight and obese patients with polycystic ovary syndrome: A randomised controlled trial. Human Reproduction. 2010;**25**:2783-2791

[14] Moran LJ, et al. Lifestyle changes in women with polycystic ovary syndrome. Cochrane Database of Systematic Reviews. 2011;**16**:2

[15] Eid GM, et al. Effective treatment of polycystic ovary syndrome with Roux-en Y gastric bypass. Surgery for Obesity and Related Diseases. 2005;**1**:77-80

[16] Teitelman M, et al. The impact of bariatric surgery on menstrual patterns. Obesity Surgery. 2006;**16**:1457-1463

[17] Malik SM, Traub ML. Defining the role of bariatric surgery in polycystic ovarian syndrome patients. World Journal of Diabetes. 2012;**3**:71-79

[18] Legro RS, et al. Effects of gastric bypass on female reproductive function. The Journal of Clinical Endocrinology & Metabolism. 2012;**97**:4540-4548

[19] Sinawat S, et al. Long versus short course treatment with metformin and clomiphene citrate for ovulation induction in women with PCOS. Cochrane Database of Systematic Reviews. 2012;**17**:10

[20] Moghetti P. Metformin effects on clinical features, endocrine and metabolic profiles. The Journal of Clinical Endocrinology and Metabolism. 2000;**85**(1):139

[21] Diamanti Kandrakis E, et al. Metformin: An old medication of new fashion: Evolving new molecular mechanisms and clinical implications in polycystic ovary syndrome. European Journal of Endocrinology. 2010;**162**:193-212

[22] Nanderpoor N, et al. Metformin and lifestyle modification in polycystic ovary syndrome: Systematic review and meta analysis. Human Reproduction Update. 2015;**21**:560-574

[23] Tang T, et al. Insulin-sensitising drugs (metformin, rosiglitazone, pioglitazone, D-chiro-inositol) for women with polycystic ovary syndrome, oligoamenorrhoea and subfertility. Cochrane Database of Systematic Reviews. 2012

[24] Palomba S, et al. Prospective parallel randomized, double-blind, double-dummy controlled clinical trial comparing clomiphene citrate and metformin as the first line treatment for ovulation induction in non-obese anovulatory women with polycystic ovary syndrome. The Journal of Clinical Endocrinology and Metabolism. 2005;**90**:4068-4074

[25] Begum MR, et al. Pre-treatment and co-administration of oral antidiabetic agent with clomiphene citrate or rFSH for ovulation induction in clomiphene-citrate-resistant polycystic ovary syndrome. Journal of Obstetrics and Gynaecology Research. 2013;**39**:966-973

[26] Bordewijk EM, et al. Metformin during ovulation induction with gonadotrophins followed by timed intercourse or intrauterine insemination for subfertility associated with polycystic ovary syndrome. Cochrane Database of Systematic Reviews. 2017;**24**:1

[27] Greenblatt RB, et al. Induction of ovulation with MRL/41. Preliminary report. JAMA. 1961;**178**:101-104

[28] Dehbashi S. Effect of clomiphene-citrate on endometria; thickness and echogenic patterns. International Journal of Gynaecology and Obstetrics. 2003;**80**(1):49

[29] Rostami-Hodjegan A. Monitoring plasma concentrations to individualise treatment with clomiphene-citrate. Fertility and Sterility. 2004;**81**:1187-1193

[30] Abu Hasim H, Foda O, Ghayaty E. Combined metformin clomiphene in clomiphene resistant ploycystic ovary syndrome: A systematic review and meta-analysis of randomized controlled trials. Acta Obstetricia et Gynecologica Scandinavica. 2015;**94**:921-930

[31] Imani B, et al. Predictors of patients remaining anovulatory during clomiphene citrate induction of ovulation in normogonadotrophic oligoamenorrheic infertility. The Journal of Clinical Endocrinology and Metabolism. 1998;**83**:2361-2365

[32] Dickey, et al. Effect of diagnosis, age, sperm quality and number of preovulatory follicles on the outcome of multiple cycles of clomiphene-citrate-intrauterine insemination. Fertility and Sterility. 2002;**78**:1088-1095

[33] Babak Imani MD, et al. A nomogram to predict the probability of live birth after clomiphene-citrate induction of ovulation in normogonadotrophic oligoamenorrheic infertility. Fertility and Sterility. 2002;**77**(1):91-97

[34] Kurachi K. Congenital malformations of newborn infants after clomiphene-induced ovulation. Fertility and Sterility. 1983;**40**(2):187

[35] Al-Fozan H. A randomised trial of letrozole versus clomiphene citrate in women undergoing superovulation. Fertility and Sterility. 2004;**82**(6):1561

[36] Franik S, Kremer JA, Nelen WL, Farquhar C. Aromatase inhibitors for subfertile women with polycystic ovary syndrome. Cochrane Database of Systematic Reviews. 2014;**24**:2

[37] Legro RS, et al. Letrozole vs clomiphene for infertility in the polycystic ovary syndrome. The New England Journal of Medicine. 2014;**371**(2):119-129

[38] Tulandi T, et al. Congenital malformations among 911 newborns conceived after infertility treatment with letrozole or clomiphene citrate. Fertility and Sterility. 2006;**85**(6):1761

[39] Homburg R, Hendriks ML, Konig TE, Anderson RA, Balen AH, Brincat M, et al. Clomifene citrate or low-dose FSH for the first-line treatment of infertile women with anovulation associated with polycystic ovary syndrome: A prospective randomized multinational study. Human Reproduction. 2012;**27**(2):468-473

[40] Calaf Alsina J, et al. Ovulation induction with a starting dose of 50IU of recombinant follicle stimulating hormone in WHO group II anovulatory women: The IO-50 study. BJOG. 2003;**110**:1072-1077

[41] Dickey RP. Strategies to reduce multiple pregnancies due to ovulation stimulation. Fertility and Sterility. 2009;**91**(1):1

[42] Amer SA, Li TC, Metwally M, Emarh M, Ledger WL. Randomised controlled trial comparing laparoscopic ovarian diathermy with clomiphene citrate as a first-line method of ovulation induction in women with polycystic ovary syndrome. Human Reproduction. 2009;**24**(1):219

[43] Farquhar C, Brown J, Marjorbanks J. Laparoscopic drilling by diathermy or laser for ovulation induction in anovulatory polycystic ovary syndrome. Cochrane Database of Systematic Reviews. 2012;**13**:6

[44] Campo S. Ovulatory cycles, pregnancy outcomes and complications after surgical treatment of polycystic ovary syndrome. Obstetrical & Gynecological Survey. 1998;**53**(5):297-308

[45] Mancini F, et al. Gonadotrophin-releasing hormone-antagonists vs long agonist in in-vitro fertilization patients with polycystic ovary syndrome: A meta-analysis. Gynecological Endocrinology. 2011;**27**(3):150-155

[46] Al-Inany HG, Abou-Setta AM, Aboulghar M. Gonadotrophin-releasing hormone antagonists for assisted conception: A Cochrane review. Reproductive Biomedicine Online. 2007;**14**(5):640-649

[47] Lin H, Li Y, Li L, Wang W, Yang D, Zhang Q. Is a GnRh antagonsist protocol better in PCOS patients? A meta-analysis of RCTs. PLoS. 2014;**18**:9(3)

[48] Levinsohn-Taror O, Friedler S, Schachter M, Raziel A, Strassburger D, Ron-El R. Coasting—What is the best formula? Hudman Reproduction. 2003;**18**(5):937

[49] Tso LO, Costello MF, Albuquerque LE, Andriolo RB, Macedo CR. Metformin treatment before and during IVF or ICSI in women with polycystic ovary syndrome. Cochrane Database of Systematic Reviews. 2014;**18**:11

[50] Palomba S, Falbo A, La Sala GB. Effects of metformin with polycystic ovary syndrome treated with gonadotrophins for in vitro fertilization and intracytoplasmic sperm injection cycles: A systematic review and meta-analysis of randomised controlled trials. BJOG. 2013;**120**(3):267

[51] Fadini R, et al. Effect of different gonadotrophin priming on IVM oocytes from women with normal ovaries: A prospective randomized study. Reproductive Biomedicine Online. 2009;**19**:343-351

[52] Walls ML, Hunter T, Ryan JP, Keelan JA, Nathan E, Hart RJ. In vitro maturation as an alternative to standard in vitro fertilization for patients diagnosed with polycystic ovaries: A comparative analysis of fresh, frozen and cumulative cycle outcomes. Human Reproduction. 2015;**30**(1):88-96

Chapter 6

Contribution of Autophagy to the Physiological and Pathophysiological Functions in the Mammalian Testis

Zonghao Tang and Zhengchao Wang

Additional information is available at the end of the chapter

http://dx.doi.org/10.5772/67878

Abstract

Mammalian spermatogenesis is a high regulated biological process occurring in the seminiferous tubules in the testis. The processing of this program requires delicate balance between cell proliferation, differentiation, apoptosis, and expedite cell interaction. Autophagy, an evolutionarily conserved cell reprograming machinery, had been shown to function as an important regulatory mechanism in spermatogenesis and steroid production in testis. Herein, we mainly focused on our understanding of autophagy in mammalian testis. By showing autophagy in physiological and pathophysiological conditions, we try to elicit the regulatory role of autophagy in spermatogenic cells and somatic cells of testis. Moreover, this review is intended to point out factors and mechanisms, which contribute to the initiation of autophagy in testicular cells.

Keywords: autophagy, physiological functions, pathophysiological functions, spermatogenesis, testis

1. Introduction

Macroautophagy (hereafter referred to as autophagy) is an evolutionarily conserved mechanism of sequestering part of cell component into cyclic processes to reverse adverse micro-environmental conditions, including limited nutrient supplies, hypoxia and some other stresses. By autophagy, misfolded proteins and impaired organelles are packaged by double membrane structure and delivered into lysosomes for cargo degrading. The basic structure of autophagosome was first revealed by Ashford and Porter [1], who described membrane-bound vacuoles in rat liver cells. As research continues, researchers observed autophagosomes in many other cell types, suggesting that autophagy is a ubiquitous mechanism in eukaryotes. Of note, autophagy is known as the only mechanism to degrade large structures, including organelles and misfolded proteins. Phylogenetically conserved role of autophagy is considered to balance the metabolic homeostasis of cell under dwindling nutrient supplies and other external perturbations. Cellular autophagic machinery induces rapid mobilization of endogenous dispensable reserves, which ensures the speedy generation of retrieving fuel for ATP synthesis [2]. Therefore, the initiation of autophagy reduces the sensitivity of cell to nutrient deprivation. In tumor cell lines, autophagy, as a mean to anti adverse microenvironment, is more prevalent than normal cells. Also, autophagy is indispensable to the survival of normal cells, and the maintenance of basal autophagy is crucial to the survival and function of many cell types in physiological settings, especially in nerve cells [3]. The abnormity of autophagy is related to many diseases such as aging, cancer, cardiac disease, and obesity.

In addition, various internal disorders and external stresses might function as initiators of autophagy such as DNA injury, toxicant exposure, heat stress, hypoxia and nutrient deprivation. Autophagy can protect the survival of cell or accelerate the process of cell apoptosis depending on the situation of cellular microenvironment. The relationship between autophagy and apoptosis has been detailedly documented in many papers [4]. However, the participation of autophagy in testicular function has received little attention in the literature. Here, we will address the consequences for testicular endocrine homeostasis and spermatogenesis in physiological and pathophysiological conditions, thereby eliciting the regulatory roles of autophagy on spermatogenic cells and somatic cells in testis.

2. The involvement of autophagy in spermatogenesis

The main testicular functions are related to endocrine secretion and the output of functional sperm. The secretion of endocrine is mainly accomplished by Leydig cells, whereas the production of mature functional sperm is initiated from so-called seminiferous tubules. During spermatogenesis, the germ cells undergo several structural reorganizations including the generation of the acrosome, the condensation of the nuclear chromatin, the rearrangement of the mitochondria, the assembly of the sperm flagella, and the removal of unnecessary cytoplasm to product functional sperm [5]. The development and differentiation of germ cells require drastic cytoskeleton remodeling, enhanced energy consuming and components degrading. For this, autophagy can "kill two birds with one stone" by eliminates needless cellular materials and providing supports for the subsequent creation of new components [6]. It had been established that autophagy is basically induced in diploid germ cells, while deeply involved in the restructure of spermatid shaping during spermiogenesis. The functional role of autophagy had demonstrated to be an indispensable mechanism for sperm production, and the deficiency of autophagy finally results in male infertility.

2.1. Autophagy in diploid germ cells

Spermatogenesis is the process that transforms spermatogonia into sperm over an extended period of time takes place in seminiferous tubule boundaries of the testis. Mammalian testicular diploid germ cells, including spermatogonia and spermatocyte, proliferate first by repeated mitotic divisions and then by meiosis to form haploid spermatids. During this period, chromosomes duplication, genetic recombination, and many other cellular meiotic accessary processes occurred ensuring that high differentiated sperm could be successfully released into the tubule lumen [7]. The activation of autophagy is crucial for the maintenance of cellular energetic balance in spermatogenic cells. In testis, spermatogonial stem cells (SSCs) are suggested as the foundation of mammalian spermatogenesis and fertility. Histologically, SSCs are rare, contributing only 0.03% of all germ cells in rodent testis [8]. Similar with the property of hematopoietic stem cells (HSCs), SSCs sustain life-long spermatogenic property. Studies had suggested that the occurrence of autophagy is essential for HSCs maintenance, and loss of autophagy lead to accumulation of mitochondria, reactive oxygen species (ROS), and DNA damage [9]. However, there are no investigations about the regulatory role of autophagy in spermatogonia. It is possible that the maintenance of cellular basal autophagy in SSCs is also a self-protective mechanism during its differentiation and self-renewing similar with that of HSCs. Noteworthy, the autophagy level of SSCs is relatively lower than other types of germ cells in testis, such as round and elongating spermatids under physiological conditions. Furthermore, the autophagy is not involved in the postnatal development of spermatogonium and spermatocyte because the absence of autophagy at spermatogonium (d7) and spermatocyte (d15) stages [10].

Under physiological conditions, high rate of cell division during spermatogenesis implies correspondingly elevated levels of mitochondrial oxygen consumption and ROS generation in spermatogonia. Mechanistically, the production of ROS is a required physiological event for the renewal of spermatogonia, the functional maturation and capacitation of spermatozoa [11]. On the other hand, ROS also participates in the induction of cellular autophagy via initiating diverse downstream signaling pathways [12, 13]. Glutathione (GSH) plays a key role in the antioxidant defense of spermatogonial cells, and high concentration of GSH has been reported in mouse testicular germ cells [14]. It had been established that GSH is involved in the regulation of autophagy in many types of cells [15, 16]. In spermatogonia, the depletion of GSH leads to the induction of autophagy. Interestingly, the depletion of GSH does not influence the level of ROS, while contributing to the downregulation of S-glutathionylated proteins, protein S-glutathionylation is initially described as a protein oxidation process, thereby leading to the induction of autophagy in spermatogonia [17]. These evidences suggest that the oxidative stress might be one of the main factors that physiologically turn on autophagy in SSCs by controlling the level of S-glutathionylated proteins in spermatogonia. Mechanistic studies suggest that GSH depletion initiates autophagy by an AMPK independent signaling pathway. The activation of autophagy induced by GSH depletion does not contribute to the alteration of energetic status in spermatogonia. It is possible that physiological fluctuation of autophagy level around the basal autophagic thresholds is accepted by germ cells.

During the initiation of autophagy, Beclin1 and p62 are two important proteins that ubiquitously implicated in the formation of autophagosomes and the recognition of autophagic cargos in many cell types. The expression of Beclin1 frequently shows similar tendency with that of LC3-II, while p62 shows opposite tendency. And, it is accepted that the expression of Beclin1 and p62 is not always consistent with expected tendency during the initiation of autophagy. However, there is a controversy about the expression of Beclin1 in spermatogonia under nutrient deprivation. As Mancilla et al. suggest that the expression of Beclin1 is not altered in nutrient starvation induced autophagy, while Wang et al. draw an opposite conclusion [18]. It is possible that inconsistent results are caused by their different starvation conditions. The activation of NF-κB pathway is recognized as the mechanism of autophagy induction in spermatogonia under nutrient deprivation. In addition, ankyrin repeat domain 49 (ANKRD49), an evolutionarily conserved protein highly expressed in testes, can significantly enhance the transcriptional activation of NF-κB, therefore upregulating autophagy level of spermatogonia under starvation [18].

Apoptosis, necrosis, and autophagy have been described as typical cell death programs. In the testis, the death of spermatocyte is crucial for controlling sperm output [19]. With this regard, apoptosis, necrosis, and autophagy are mechanistically related machineries in spermatocyte for the control of testicular homeostasis. Under physiological conditions, the death of spermatocyte is associated with available energy supply. It has been documented that spermatocytes use lactate rather than glucose as their primary substrate for the production of ATP [20]. In vitro studies revealed that after 6 h of culture a significant increase of cell death is detected for spermatocytes cultured in glucose, while there is no significant increase in cells cultured with lactate. However, autophagy levels are significantly increased in spermatocytes cultured with glucose or lactate after 12 and 24 h, suggesting that autophagy might function as a pro-death role in rat spermatocytes under certain metabolic conditions [21]. In spermatocyte, the molecular mechanism is not yet clear about what factors determine whether autophagy acts as a cytoprotective defender or a cytotoxic trigger and whether cytotoxicity occurs as the result of self-cannibalism, the specific degradation of cytoprotective factors, or other as of yet undefined mechanisms [22]. It is certain that autophagy is not involved in the regulation of spermatocyte in newly born infant, because the expression of autophagic marker proteins is absent from spermatocytes at postnatal day 15 [23]. However, the physiological roles of autophagy in spermatocyte of adult mice still remain unknown.

Relatively, the autophagy levels of both spermatogonia and spermatocyte are maintained at a low level compared with other types of germ cell in mammalian testis under physiological conditions. It is established that the autophagy level is high related to inner cell status and outer microenvironments. In testis, the nutrition status of germ cells is directly associated with their mother cells, Sertoli cells. And, except for the early phase of spermatogenesis from type B spermatogonia up to preleptotene and leptotene spermatocytes, the entire process of germ cell development is isolated from the systemic circulation because of the blood-testis barrier (BTB) created by tight junctions (TJ) between Sertoli cells near the basal lamina [24, 25]. Thus, it is clear that spermatogonia and spermatocytes are suffered to different physiological environments. The difference of physiological hormonal subjection might be one of the main factors that led to the inhibition of autophagy in diploid germ cells. In testis, follicle-stimulating hormone (FSH) in all cycles is to increase spermatogonia and subsequent spermatocyte numbers, which is similar to the physiological role of FSH on granulosal cells. Previous studies had demonstrated that FSH functions as an autophagy inhibitor in ovarian granulosal cells [26]. We hypothesis that FSH might also contribute to the inhibition of autophagy in testicular diploid germ cells, while detailed molecular pathways in diploid germ cells still remain to be documented.

2.2. The role of autophagy and spermatid differentiation

Spermiogenesis is a sophisticated and highly ordered spermatid differentiation process that requires reorganization of cellular structures and readjustment of cellular physiological functions. The successful removal of cytoplasm is thought to be critical for the generation of functional and motile spermatozoa. The dysfunction of spermatozoa is mainly caused by the abnormal of spermatozoa head or the coil of its flagellum. Autophagy is deeply involved in the processes of spermatozoa formation, and the deficiency of autophagy leads to various spermatozoa defects, which could be classified into three groups, the abnormal of spermatozoa head, the coil of spermatozoa tail, and the aggregate of spermatozoa [23]. For the spermatozoa with bent head, a large portion of cytoplasm is remained connecting the bent head and the tail, thus lead to the inhibition of its beating. For the spermatozoa with coiled tail, the sperm tail is seriously coiled with mislocalized and poorly condensed mitochondria, while aggregated spermatozoa is characterized by the presence of clustered sperm tails and is wrapped by membrane and some cytoplasm.

In spermatozoa, the acrosome is a specialized membranous organelle located over the anterior part of the sperm nucleus, which is important for the dispersion of cumulus cells and the penetration of the zona pellucida of the oocyte during fertilization. The formation of acrosome involves the reprogramming of cellular cytoskeleton, which requiring the induction of autophagy to assist the rearrangement of cellular cytoskeleton. Indeed, comparing with diploid germ cells, the expression of autophagy-related proteins such as LC3 and Atg7 are significantly higher in elongated spermatid. Furthermore, the expression of LC3 could be observed firstly in round spermatid (d20) of postnatal testis, which indicating the involvement of autophagy in early testicular spermatid development. Ablation of autophagy by germ cell-specific knockout of Atg7 leads to the decrease of testicular weight, the detachment of premature germ cells, and the malformation of spermatozoa, which significantly reduce the fertility of male mice [10]. Particularly, many spermatozoa from Atg7−/− mice are endowed with irregularly shaped round heads similar to human globozoospermia, a severe fertility disorder characterized by round-headed spermatozoa with malformed acrosome or without acrosome at all. In addition, the deficiency of Atg7 also leads to many other acrosomal defects, such as the mis-localization, the deformation and the fragmentation of spermatozoal acrosome; thus, they failed to acquire the typical crescent moon shape [10].

The formation of acrosome is grouped into four phases: Golgi, Cap, Acrosome, and Maturation [27]. Autophagy participates in acrosome biogenesis starting in the Golgi phase. In normal conditions, Golgi apparatus-derived proacrosomal vesicles are fused into a single acrosomal vesicle attached to one end of the nucleus in the Golgi-phase spermatids. After Atg7 disruption, multiple small vesicles of the Golgi-phase spermatids are failed to fuse with each other, thereby showing multiple acrosomal structures. In cap phase, 10% of the spermatids had multi acrosomal vesicles or aggregates, and the accumulation of proacrosomal vesicles derived from the Golgi apparatus leads to the shrinkage of acrosome [10]. These evidences suggest that the malformation of acrosomes most likely caused by the failure of proacrosomal vesicles to fuse and be transported to the preacrosome at one end of the nuclei. Mechanistically, the function of Atg7 in acrosome biogenesis might be similar to its role in autophagy induction. Within autophagy, LC3-lipid conjugation is a reversible process, LC3 residing on the outer face of the vesicle can be recycled by Atg4, whereas LC3 on the inner surface is ultimately degraded. In spermatid, LC3 is only colocalized with the trans-Golgi network marker TGN38 rather than the acrosome maker sp56. Therefore, membrane-associated LC3 might participate in the fusion of Golgi apparatus-derived proacrosomal vesicles and their transportation to the acrosome. After fusion with the acrosome, LC3 will be either recycled or degraded. After Atg7 disruption, LC3 is failed to colocalize with TGN38, causing the accumulation of proacrosomal vesicles in the concave region near the trans-Golgi stacks [10]. Finally, this accumulation impairs the increase in acrosome volume in the later stages, whereupon resulting in defective acrosome formation.

A mammalian spermatozoon is characterized by two morphological and functional components; the head and the flagellum, both parts are optimized for special tasks. The formation of spermatozoa head and flagellum requires the mobilization and specialization of cytoskeleton in spermatid. During this process, autophagy is extensively involved in the regulation and the remolding of cell shapes by altering cellular cytoskeletons [28]. In round and elongating spermatids, autophagy is recognized as a potent regulator of cell structures in both types of germ cells. It has been established that except for the role of autophagy on acrosome shaping, it is also involved in the formation of sperm flagella via the rearrangement of the mitochondria and the elimination of unnecessary cytoplasm to facilitate spermatozoa motility. Gene knockout corroborated the role of autophagy in spermiogenesis. As mice spermatids begin to elongate from step 8, the deficiency of Atg7 makes no change on spermatids before step 8 [10].

PDLIM1 (PDZ and LIM domain protein 1) is a member of the PDZ and LIM protein family, containing an N-terminal PDZ domain and a C-terminal LIM domain. It is acknowledged that PDLIM1 acts as a scaffold to bring other proteins to the cytoskeleton and is also involved in cytoskeleton reorganization in many types of cells [29, 30]. During spermiogenesis, PDLIM1 functions as a mediator between autophagy and cytoskeleton organization. Under normal conditions, the degradation of PDLIM1 by the autophagy-lysosome pathway is needed to maintain a proper dynamics of the cytoskeleton network whereupon assuring that spermatids differentiation could be processed smoothly. The disruption of autophagy results in failure engulf of PDLIM1 by autophagosomes, thereby leading to their accumulation in the cytoplasm. The accumulation of PDLIM1 disrupts the proper dynamics of the cytoskeleton and finally leads to the inefficient cytoplasm removal during spermiogenesis. In normal testis, F-actin signal is stronger than PDLIM1 in the elongating spermatids, and also, F-actin based acroplaxome provides a docking site for the acrosome development, thus anchors it to the spermatid nucleus [31]. Autophagy impairment strongly increases the level of PDLIM1 in spermatids and disrupts the organization of cytoskeleton, thus leading to the disorganization of flagellar "9+2" structure and other cytoskeletal components in spermatozoa [23]. The well organization of spermatozoal flagellum is crucial to the normal motility of spermatozoa, while the deficiency of autophagy significantly changed sperm motility parameters including the average path velocity (VAP), straight-line velocity (VSL), and curvilinear velocity (VCL).

In round spermatids, autophagy is also involved in the degradation of other cellular components. Among which, the degradation of chromatoid body has been recently uncovered. In germ cells, the chromatoid body (CB) is an unusually large germ granule, which is initially formed in the cytoplasm of late pachytene spermatocytes. After meiosis, CB is condensed to its final form and maintain a distinct cytoplasmic feature throughout the differentiation of round spermatids [32]. During the elongation of spermatids, the size of CB will be shrink forming a ring around the base of the flagellum [33]. The accessary material from the CB is finally discarded together with the rest of the cytoplasm in the residual body. It is demonstrated that the clearance of these materials is mainly undertook by autophagy via an FYCO1-dependent pathway, and the induction of autophagy enables the homeostasis of CB [34]. Mechanistically, FYCO1 functions as a docking site for LC3 and LAMP1-positive membranes mediating the recruitment of autophagosome and lysosome to the CB. In addition, an intriguing option is that some specific RNA species are also eliminated via FYCO1-mediated autophagy [35]. However, the disruption of FYCO1 pathway in round spermatid somewhat does not impair the fertility of male.

3. Autophagy and the functions of testicular somatic cells

Leydig cells and Sertoli cells are two types of somatic cells exist in mammalian testis. Histologically, Leydig cell and Sertoli cells share different locations in testis, which implies diverse hormonal exposure and different physiological functions. Both types of testicular somatic cells adopt autophagy as a regulatory mechanism for the maintenance of cellular homeostasis. During spermatogenesis, physiological orders are assigned to each seminiferous tubule, and seminiferous tubule substantially acts as a functional unit of testis. Leydig cells are histologically localized in the interval of seminiferous tubules, while it also exerted in the regulation of spermatogenesis by secreting testosterone. In addition to the role of testosterone on germ cells, some of the cellular biological programs are also selectively regulated by testosterone via an autophagy-dependent pathway in Sertoli cells. Comparatively, the Sertoli cells maintain tight contact with germ cells in seminiferous tubules. In essence, the functions of Sertoli cells are related to its paralleled structural basis, the malformation of cellular structure frequently leads to the infertility of male. Autophagy plays pivotal roles in the regulation of Sertoli cell functions via cytoskeleton adjustment [36].

3.1. Autophagy and Leydig cell function

Previous researchers had revealed the regulatory roles of autophagy in steroid production and secretion [37]. In male mammal, testis contributes about 95% of total circulating testosterone, and Leydig cell is the primary testosterone contributor in mammalian testis. Testosterone is necessary for male fetal sexual differentiation, adult secondary sex characteristics maintenance, and spermatogenesis. Like many other types of steroid-producing cells, Leydig cells are typically own enlarged mitochondria than other cell types. The production of steroid is an energy-intensive engineering, which directly related to the damage of mitochondrial function. The involvement of autophagy in cellular organelle degradation had been reported in other cell types [38]. It has demonstrated that the relative frequency of autophagy in Leydig cells is higher than many other cell types [39]. Consistently, abundant autophagosome engulfed organelles are also observed in rat Leydig cells, most of the organelles enclosed in the autophagic vacuoles are SER and mitochondria, organelles that involved in the production of androgens. These evidences lead to the hypothesis that the autophagic activity might relate to the regulation of hormonal secretion in Leydig cells. Indeed, the process of autophagy is high related to the production of testosterone in rat Leydig cells, and the deficiency of autophagy is frequently associated with the dysregulation of testicular homeostasis [40]. However, little is known about the relationship between autophagy and testosterone production in Leydig cells under physiological conditions.

It is acknowledged that autophagy is a predominant cytoprotective rather than a self-destructive process in normal cells [41]. Accordingly, autophagy is involved in mediating protective effects in multiple rodent models of organ damage affecting the heart, liver, nervous system, and kidney. Reduced autophagy level has been associated with accelerated aging process, while promote autophagy could partially protect cell from natural aging process [42]. The induction of autophagy is also involved in the maintenance of testosterone level in rat testis. In the old rat, the accumulation of ROS is significantly increased comparing with that of young rat. ROS act as one of the main factors that lead to the downregulation of StAR (steroidogenic acute regulatory protein) protein level and the secretion of testosterone by activating p38 mitogen-activated protein kinase or c-Jun [43]. In Leydig cells, autophagy regulates the accumulation of ROS by promoting the clearance of damaged mitochondria, oxidized cellular substrates, and by activating antioxidant systems. Inhibition of autophagy by disrupting Beclin1 decreases the expression of StAR, while inducing autophagy in Leydig cells from aged or young rat by rapamycin increases the expression of StAR under the stimulation of LH [40]. Thus, it is possible that the downregulation of testosterone in aged Leydig cells might result from two aspects: (1) the deficiency of autophagic machinery and (2) the increase of ROS level. However, the increase in ROS could also be attributed to the compromise of autophagic efficiency.

Endocytosis is an active transport machinery, by which a cell transports molecules and proteins into the cell by engulfing them in an energy-using process [44]. Similar with the function of autophagy, endocytic mechanism plays an important role in regulating how cells interact with their environments. Both endocytosis and autophagy are the major pathways for transporting materials to lysosomes in animal cells, the former being responsible for uptake of extracellular constituents while the latter for degradation of cytoplasmic components. In the Leydig cells, the endocytosis remains close cooperation with autophagy whereupon leading to the degradation of respective contents. It had been shown that late endosomes deliver their endocytosed contents and lysosomal enzymes to the early autophagosomes, implying that the endocytosis and autophagy are seamlessly connected in rat Leydig cells. The collaboration of both mechanisms is efficiently mobilized in Leydig cells under physiological conditions. Different with other cell types, rat Leydig cells morphologically show typical autophagy-related morphologies, as the early signs of autophagy, called preautophagosomes, can be easily observed in the ultrastructure of Leydig cells, while these structures are rarely shown in other normal cell types even when autophagy is induced [45].

http://dx.doi.org/10.5772/67878

3.2. Autophagy is required for structural modulation in Sertoli cell

During spermiogenesis, the differentiating germ cells undergo a successive morphological transformation from round spermatids to sperm, which requires cellular remodeling of spermatids and the assistance of Sertoli cells. The Sertoli cell is involved in the degradation of many useless components within seminiferous tubule, such as spermatid residual bodies (RB) and the apoptotic germ cells. Sertoli cell has a prominent ability to metabolize those phagocytized materials. In testis, the homeostatic phagocytosis of Sertoli cells varies depending on seminiferous epithelium cycle and reaching its maximum during spermiation [46]. In Sertoli cells, both autophagy and phagocytosis may undertake similar mission under certain circumstance, especially once a phagocytic vesicle has entered a cell. Numerous evidences had suggested that autophagy is associated with the process of phagocytosis and is atypically implicated in the degradation of external substrates entering via phagocytosis in Sertoli cells [47]. Generally, blood-separated tissues use their tissue specific nonprofessional phagocytes for homeostatic phagocytosis [48]. In the testis, Sertoli cells manage illegitimate substrates and legitimate substrates with different pathways. Exposing of cultured Sertoli cells to either illegitimate (such as photoreceptor outer segments generated from other tissue) or legitimate substrates (such as residue body generated by differentiating germ cell), both substrate types are ingested by phagocytosis. Nevertheless, autophagy is selectively involved in the degradation of those illegitimate substrates in Sertoli cells, and the inhibition of autophagy significantly retarded the degradation of illegitimate substrates [47].

Sertoli cells play pivotal roles in the regulation of spermatogenesis by providing structural support and nourishment to developing germ cells, controlling the self-renewal and differentiation of spermatogonial stem cells (SSCs), protecting the autoreactive immune response of germ cells, and releasing spermatids at spermiation [49]. In the seminiferous epithelium, functional cell interconnections are maintained by Sertoli-Sertoli cell and Sertoli-germ cell junctions [50]. The Sertoli cell ectoplasmic specialization (ES) and the spermatid-containing acrosome-acroplaxome-manchette complex are two cytoskeletal structures that play important roles in the shaping of sperm head [51]. Among which, the ectoplasmic specialization (ES) is composed by two components, an actin-based atypical adherens junction between adjacent Sertoli cells at the blood-testis barrier (BTB) termed as basal ES, whereas between Sertoli cells and spermatids near the luminal surface of the tubule termed as apical ES [52]. The basal ES function as an important component of the blood-testis barrier (BTB) [53, 54] and apical ES (aES) interacts with the acrosome of the elongating spermatid and mechanically assists the shaping of spermatid head [50]. The function of apical ES is also related to the movement of spermatid cell and the release of the matured spermatozoa during spermiation. Successively, transportation of developing germ cells across the seminiferous epithelium is important for the processes of spermatogenesis, which requires the dynamic restructuring of ES in the epithelial cycle [23, 55, 56]. It has been demonstrated that autophagy is involved in the regulation of ES. The deficiency of autophagy by Atg7 or Atg5 ablation disturbs the assembly of both apical ES and basal

ES in the seminiferous epithelium. Mechanistic studies revealed that similar with that of spermatid, autophagy disruption impairs the degradation of PDLIM1 thereby resulting in its accumulation in Sertoli cells. Therefore, the organization of cytoskeleton in Sertoli cells is perturbed. PDLIM1 might be the primary substrate of the autophagy to regulate cytoskeleton organization, because the proper organization of the cytoskeletal structure could be significantly restored by knockdown of Pdlim1 gene in autophagy-deficient Sertoli cells. Successful organization of cytoskeleton in Sertoli cell is highly related to the produce of functional spermatozoa. The accumulation of PDLIM1 disrupts the F-actin hoops of the apical ES and related microtubule-based structures in the seminiferous epithelium, which ultimately leading to the disruption of Sertoli cell-germ cell communication thereafter contributing to the malformation of sperm head [36].

However, although autophagy plays pivotal roles in apical ES formation as well as basal ES assembling, it is not exert in the assembly of tubular and bulbous structures of TBCs (tubulobulbar complexes). In Sertoli cells, TBCs are located on both Sertoli-Sertoli cells and Sertoli cell-spermatids interface and are implicated in the restructure of ES, excess spermatid cytoplasm removing and spermatid acrosome shaping [57]. The cytoskeletal remolding of TBCs is also important to the release of sperm and the translocation of spermatocytes. Unwanted distribution of TBCs directly impaired the function of Sertoli cells as well as the communication between Sertoli cells and germ cells. Liu et al. suggested that the different influences of autophagy on apical ES and TBCs assembly might come from their different F-actin arrangements, because F-actin is packed in hexagonal arrays in the ES, while it appears as an embranchment surrounding the tubular portion of TBCs [36, 58, 59]. Furthermore, the incorrect distribution of TBCs might also be resulted from the abnormal structure of apical ES or the malformation of sperm head, whereas these possibilities still remain to be uncovered by further experimental data. Interestingly, the marker proteins that implicated in SSCs self-renewal or meiosis show no changes after the disruption of autophagy in Sertoli cells, implying that autophagy is dispensable in the self-renewing of SSCs and meiosis process of germ cells.

Androgen-binding protein (ABP) is a kind of sex hormone-binding globulin (SHBG) produced by testicular Sertoli cells, which specifically binds to and reduce the lipotropism of testosterone or dihydrotestosterone, making them more concentrated in the seminiferous tubules. High concentration of ABP is required for the process of spermatogenesis in the seminiferous tubules and the maturation of sperm maturation in the epididymis. In mammal, the production and the secretion of ABP are regulated by FSH, oestradiol, and testosterone [60–62]. In Sertoli cells, testosterone participates in the synthesis and the secretion of ABP by autophagy. In vitro studies suggest that ABP is colocalized with LC3 in primary rat Sertoli cells, and inhibition, or stimulation of autophagy considerably change both the expression pattern and level of ABP in Sertoli cells without affecting the expression of ABP mRNA, implying that the regulatory role of autophagy on the degradation of ABP is only works on its protein level. Furthermore, the inhibitory function of testosterone on autophagy is also influenced by testosterone concentrations, as enhanced concentration of testosterone further inhibits autophagic pathway [63]. Importantly, although hypoxia exposure further enhances the autophagy level of Sertoli cells, but hypoxia-induced autophagy does not change the expression of ABP in rat primary Sertoli cells, suggesting that the degradation of ABP is independent of hypoxia-induced autophagy.

4. Autophagy and testicular toxicology

The process of spermatogenesis requires well-balanced germ cell proliferation, differentiation, and death in the testis [64, 65]. However, this process can be disturbed by several endogenous or exogenous factors, including withdraw of gonadotropin or testosterone, chemical insults, heat stress, and radiation exposure. Cell apoptosis and autophagy are two major morphologically distinctive forms of programmed cell death (PCD) that play crucial roles in the development and the control of male reproductive functions. The crosstalk between autophagy and apoptosis is sophisticated in the sense that they might act synergistically or antagonistically with each other in the process of cell life and death. The normal operation of autphagic process is related to many physiological functions, whereas the dysfunction of autophagy leads to numerous diseases in human. In testis, evidences have demonstrated that autophagy plays important roles in testicular pathologies caused by oxidative stress, heat stress, toxicant exposure, and radiation exposure.

4.1. Autophagy and testicular homeostasis

Ample of evidences has documented the correlation between toxicant exposure and germ cell death. It is well known that cell may activate self-protective mechanisms in response to exogenous insults, such as chemical exposure. The activation of autophagy is important to the maintenance of cellular functions and may partially rescue the dysfunction of tissue homeostasis under adverse environments [66]. Chemical exposure is high related to the out control of tissue homeostasis. Exposure of testis to toxicants frequently leads to the activation of autophagy by different signaling pathways. Exposing testis to BPA (Bisphenol A) leads to the activation of oxidative stress, which activates autophagy mainly by inhibiting mTOR signaling pathway. Meanwhile, the phosphorylation of AMPKa and the expression of p53 might act as a contributor to the upregulation of autophagy under BPA exposure. Of note, the expression of Beclin1 is not upregulated accompany by autophagy in testis under BPA exposure [67]. With NaF exposure, the autophagy is abnormally increased as evidenced by the synchronized increase of p62, suggesting that NaF exposure impairs autophagic machinery and result in the accumulation of autophagosomes in testis [68]. In addition, autophagy is also involved in the regulation of testicular homeostasis under other toxicant treatments, for example, see Ref. [69]. As testis is composed by germ cells and somatic cells, many studies specifically evaluated the involvement of autophagy in germ cells or somatic cell to elucidate the mechanisms and functions of autophagy under specific conditions.

4.2. Autophagy and germ cell injuries

Autophagy is referred to as programmed cell death type 2, the process of which might be excessively induced under stresses, and the abnormal induction of autophagy is high related to cellular apoptosis especially under severe adverse conditions. It has been established that testicular heating can disturb spermatogenesis and cause subfertility, some testis-related diseases including cryptorchidism are also linked to testicular heating, in which the testis is exposed to body temperature rather than scrotal temperature, whereupon lead to abnormal testis function and damaged spermatogenesis in these settings [70, 71]. Autophagy is recognized as one of the regulatory factors that participate in the death of heat-treated somatic cells [72]. Similarly, heat treatment on mouse testis could also upregulate the induction of apoptosis and autophagy in the germ cells. Meanwhile, prolonged exposure time increases apoptosis as well as autophagy levels of germ cells in mouse testis. In vitro experiments corroborated the induction of autophagy in spermatocyte by heart stress. Functionally, autophagy functions as an apoptotic inducer rather than a self-protective mechanism in germ cells, because the inhibition of autophagy markedly reduces the apoptotic rate of germ cells in the testis [73].

In addition to triggering cellular dysfunction, autophagy also functions as a cytoprotective response in germ cells under stressful conditions. When treating GC-2 cell with dibutyl phthalate (DPB) significantly induces ER stress in GC-2 cells. However, the expression of caspase-12 or the phosphorylation of JNK or p38 is not changed at the indicated DBP doses, and the inhibition of ER stress increases DBP-induced GC-2 cell apoptosis. Autophagy is participated in the regulation of ER stress, because the inhibition of autophagy significantly aggravated apoptosis. In vivo study indicates that autophagy is consistently induced in rat testis under DBP exposure. The suppression of ER stress or autophagy aggravates DBP-induced injury in rat testis, as evidenced by the greater reduction in testicular index and decrease in germ cells in the seminiferous tubules [74]. Except for exempting germ cells from toxicant insults, autophagy also plays vital roles in germ cells under the exposure of some physical factors. Studies had demonstrated that exposure of spermatocytes to radiofrequency (RF) can lead to the accumulation of intracellular ROS and thereafter inducing autophagy through the activation of ERK signaling pathway. However, the activation of autophagy can dwindle the accumulation of ROS within spermatocytes. Therefore, the induction of autophagy is an indispensable mechanism for germ cell survival [75].

4.3. Functions of autophagy in testicular somatic cell impairment

In addition to the involvement of autophagy in germ cells, studies also evaluated the role of autophagy in testicular somatic cell under toxicant exposure. It had been revealed that exposure of rat Leydig cells to zearalenone (ZEA) leads to the induction of autophagy in Leydig cell. The induction of autophagy is related to the concentration of ZEA, as the expression of LC3-II is peaked at 5 μg/mL and then gradually decreased. In Leydig cells, the activation of autophagy acts as a cytoprotective role in ZEA-treated Leydig cells. Inhibition of autophagy markedly increases the apoptosis level of Leydig cells compared with that of ZEA treatment alone. By contrast, the apoptosis level decreased after the cotreatment of ZEA and rapamycin [76].

Sertoli cells (SCs) orchestrate the processes of spermatogenesis by nourishing and adapting environment for germ cell survival and differentiation. Toxicant-induced dysregulation of SCs leads to the reduction in its supportive capacity, thus impairing spermatogenesis and fertility. Studies had revealed that exposure of SCs to 4-Nonylphenol (NP) leads to the upregulation of ROS level, which in turn activates JNK signaling pathway and mediates the induction of JNK-dependent autophagy [77]. Functionally, autophagy acts as a self-protective machinery in SCs under NP treatment, because the inhibition of autophagy considerably increases the level of cell death [78]. Obviously, the abnormal induction of autophagy in SCs under toxicant exposure is also related to the process of apoptosis. For example, see Ref. [79].

5. Concluding remarks

The available data suggest that autophagy is deeply involved in the regulation of testicular homeostasis. For example, autophagy is exerted in the regulation of germ cell survival, the transformation of spermatids, the rearrangement of Sertoli cells, and the testosterone production of Leydig cells (**Table 1**). In mammal, the orchestrated cooperation of germ cells and somatic cells is required for the production of functional sperm. During spermatogenesis, the induction of autophagy is an indispensable mechanism for the paralleled structural transformation of spermatids and Sertoli cells, ensuring that acrosome and flagellum could be successively established. However, it is necessary to illuminate the regulatory roles of hormones such as testosterone, luteinizing hormone (LH), and FSH on the function of autophagy in germ cells under physiological and pathological conditions. It is noteworthy that the decline in fertility result from environmental exposure has caught the worldwide attention recently. Evidences had uncovered that the exposure of testis or cultured testicular cells to adverse environments prompted the initiation of autophagy in both germ cells and somatic cells. However, there is short of relevant data about the regulatory role of autophagy in testicular-related diseases. Most of relevant data are toxicant exposure related, which could not accurately reflect the involvements of autophagy in pathological conditions. It is then the topic of what the optima strategy would be to utilize autophagy to remove deleterious side effects whereupon bring benefits to the therapy of infertility and many other testis related disease.

Cell types	Roles of autophagy	Related dysfunctions
Diploid germ cells	Function as an adaptive response	Germ cell death
Spermatid	Regulation of acrosome and flagellum formation	Sperm head malformation; reduction of sperm motility
Leydig cell	Maintenance of testosterone production	Reduction in testosterone aging
Sertoli cell	Regulation of the formation of ectoplasmic specialization Regulation of tubulobulbar complexes distribution Regulation of androgen-binding protein half-life	Dysregulation of apical ES basal ES perturbation Disorder of Sertoli cell cytoskeleton structure Prolonged ABP half-life

Table 1. Physiological and pathological roles of autophagy in the mammalian testis.

Acknowledgements

This study was supported by National Natural Science Foundation of China (31271255), Fujian Provincial Natural Science Foundation (2016J01145) and Fujian Province Science and Technology Project of The Education Department (JAT160118 and JZ160426).

Author details

Zonghao Tang and Zhengchao Wang*

*Address all correspondence to: zcwang@fjnu.edu.cn

Provincial Key Laboratory for Developmental Biology and Neurosciences, College of Life Sciences, Fujian Normal University, Fuzhou, PR China

References

[1] Ashford TP, Porter KR. Cytoplasmic components in hepatic cell lysosomes. Journal of Cell Biology. 1962;**12**(12):198. doi:10.1083/jcb.12.1.198

[2] Singh R, Cuervo AM. Autophagy in the cellular energetic balance. Cell Metabolism. 2011;**13**(5):495-504. doi:10.1016/j.cmet.2011.04.004

[3] Kuma A, Hatano M, Matsui M, Yamamoto A, Nakaya H, Yoshimori T, et al. The role of autophagy during the early neonatal starvation period. Nature. 2004;**432**(7020):1032-1036. doi:10.1038/nature03029

[4] Thorburn A. Apoptosis and autophagy: regulatory connections between two supposedly different processes. Apoptosis. 2008;**13**(1):1-9. doi:10.1007/s10495-007-0154-9

[5] Lalli M, Clermont Y. Structural changes of the head components of the rat spermatid during late spermiogenesis. Developmental Dynamics. 1981;**160**(4):419-434. doi:10.1002/aja.1001600406

[6] Mizushima N, Levine B. Autophagy in mammalian development and differentiation. Nature Cell Biology. 2010;**12**(9):823-830. doi:10.1038/ncb0910-823

[7] De Kretser DM, Loveland KL, Meinhardt A, Simorangkir D, Wreford N. Spermatogenesis. Human Reproduction. 1998;**13**(1):1-8. doi:10.1093/humrep/13.suppl_1.1

[8] Tagelenbosch RAJ, Rooij DGD. A quantitative study of spermatogonial multiplication and stem cell renewal in the C3H/101 F 1 hybrid mouse. Mutation Research/Fundamental & Molecular Mechanisms of Mutagenesis. 1993;**290**(2):193-200. doi:10.1016/0027-5107(93)90159-D

[9] Mortensen M, Soilleux EJ, Djordjevic G, Tripp R, Lutteropp M, Sadighiakha E, et al. The autophagy protein Atg7 is essential for hematopoietic stem cell maintenance. The Journal of Experimental Medicine. 2011;**208**(3):455-467. doi:10.1084/jem.20101145

[10] Shang Y, Wang H, Jia P, Zhao H, Liu C, Liu W, et al. Autophagy regulates spermatid differentiation via degradation of PDLIM1. Autophagy. 2016;**12**(9):1575-1592. doi:10.1080/15548627.2016.1192750

[11] Morimoto H, Iwata K, Ogonuki N, Inoue K, Atsuo O, Kanatsushinohara M, et al. ROS are required for mouse spermatogonial stem cell self-renewal. Cell Stem Cell. 2013;**12**(6):774-786. doi:10.1016/j.stem.2013.04.001

[12] Ding W, Ni H, Li M, Liao Y, Chen X, Stolz DB, et al. Nix is critical to two distinct phases of mitophagy: reactive oxygen species (ROS)-mediated autophagy induction and Parkin-ubiqutin-p62-mediated mitochondria priming. Journal of Biological Chemistry. 2010;**285**(36):27879-27890. doi:10.1074/jbc.M110.119537

[13] Wang Y, Nartiss Y, Steipe B, Mcquibban GA, Kim PKM. ROS-induced mitochondrial depolarization initiates PARK2/PARKIN-dependent mitochondrial degradation by autophagy. Autophagy. 2012;**8**(10):1462-1476. doi:10.4161/auto.21211

[14] Grosshans K, Calvin HI. Estimation of glutathione in purified populations of mouse testis germ cells. Biology of Reproduction. 1986;**33**(5):1197-1205. doi:10.1095/biolreprod33.5.1197

[15] Desideri E, Filomeni G, Ciriolo MR. Glutathione participates in the modulation of starvation-induced autophagy in carcinoma cells. Autophagy. 2012;**8**(12):1769-1781. doi:10.4161/auto.22037

[16] Itoh T, Ohguchi K, Nozawa Y, Akao Y. Intracellular glutathione regulates sesquiterpene lactone-induced conversion of autophagy to apoptosis in human leukemia HL60 cells. Anticancer Research. 2009;**29**(4):1449-1457. doi:10.1503/cmaj.091016

[17] Mancilla H, Maldonado R, Cereceda K, Villarroelespíndola F, Montes dOM, Angulo C, et al. Glutathione depletion induces spermatogonial cell autophagy. Journal of Cellular Biochemistry. 2015;**116**(10):2283-2292. doi:10.1002/jcb.25178

[18] Wang H, Fan S, Pang M, Liu Y, Guo M, Liang J, et al. The ankyrin repeat domain 49 (ANKRD49) augments autophagy of serum-starved GC-1 cells through the NF-κB pathway. PLoS One. 2015;**10**(6):e0128551. doi:10.1371/journal.pone.0128551

[19] Knudson CM, Tung KS, Tourtellotte WG, Brown GA, Korsmeyer SJ. Bax-deficient mice with lymphoid hyperplasia and male germ cell death. Science. 1995;**270**(5233):96-99. doi:10.1126/science.270.5233.96

[20] Grootegoed JA, Jansen R, Hj VDM. The role of glucose, pyruvate and lactate in ATP production by rat spermatocytes and spermatids. Biochimica et Biophysica Acta. 1984;**767**(2):248-256. doi:10.1016/0005-2728(84)90194-4

[21] Bustamante-Marin X, Quiroga C, Lavandero S, Reyes JG, Moreno RD. Apoptosis, necrosis and autophagy are influenced by metabolic energy sources in cultured rat spermatocytes. Apoptosis. 2012;**17**(6):539-550. doi:10.1007/s10495-012-0709-2

[22] Levine B. Autophagy in the pathogenesis of disease. Cell. 2008;**132**(1):27-42. doi:10.1016/j.cell.2007.12.018

[23] Wang H, Wan H, Li X, Liu W, Chen Q, Wang Y, et al. Atg7 is required for acrosome biogenesis during spermatogenesis in mice. Cell Research. 2014;**24**(7):852-869. doi:10.1038/cr.2014.70

[24] Cheng CY, Mruk DD. Cell junction dynamics in the testis: Sertoli-germ cell interactions and male contraceptive development. Physiological Reviews. 2002;**82**(4):825-874. doi:10.1152/physrev.00009.2002

[25] O'Shaughnessy PJ. Hormonal control of germ cell development and spermatogenesis. Seminars in Cell & Developmental Biology. 2014;**29**(3):55-65. doi:10.1016/j.semcdb.2014.02.010

[26] Choi JY, Jo MW, Lee EY, Yoon BK, Choi DS. The role of autophagy in follicular development and atresia in rat granulosa cells. Fertility and Sterility. 2010;**93**(8):2532-2537. doi:10.1016/j.fertnstert.2009.11.021

[27] Berruti G, Paiardi C. Acrosome biogenesis. Spermatogenesis. 2011;**1**(2):95-98. doi:10.4161/spmg.1.2.16820

[28] Mostowy S, Cossart P. Autophagy and the cytoskeleton. Autophagy. 2011;**7**(7):780-782. doi:10.4161/auto.7.7.15593

[29] Vallenius T, Luukko K, Mäkelä TP. CLP-36 PDZ-LIM protein associates with nonmuscle alpha-actinin-1 and alpha-actinin-4. J Biol Chem. 2000 Apr 14; **275**(15): 11100-5. PMID: 10753915

[30] Miehe U, Kadyrov M, Neumaier-Wagner P, Bartz C, Rath W, Huppertz B. Expression of the actin stress fiber-associated protein CLP36 in the human placenta. Histochemistry and Cell Biology. 2006;**126**(4):465-471. doi:10.1007/s00418-006-0182-5

[31] Kierszenbaum AL, Tres LL, Rivkin E, Kang-Decker N, van Deursen JM. The acroplaxome is the docking site of Golgi-derived myosin Va/Rab27a/b- containing proacrosomal vesicles in wild-type and Hrb mutant mouse spermatids. Biology of Reproduction. 2004;**70**(5):1400-1410. doi:10.1095/biolreprod.103.025346

[32] Walt H, Armbruster BL. Actin and RNA are components of the chromatoid bodies in spermatids of the rat. Cell and Tissue Research. 1984;**236**(2):487-490. doi:10.1007/BF00214254

[33] Fawcett DW, Eddy EM, Phillips DM. Observations on the fine structure and relationships of the chromatoid body in mammalian spermatogenesis. Biology of Reproduction. 1970;**2**(1):129-153. doi:10.1095/biolreprod2.1.129

[34] Da Ros M, Lehtiniemi T, Olotu O, et al. FYCO1 and autophagy control the integrity of the haploid male germ cell-specific RNP granules. Autophagy. Forthcoming. doi:10.1080/15548627.2016.1261319

[35] Guo H, Chitiprolu M, Gagnon D, Meng L, Pereziratxeta C, Lagace D, et al. Autophagy supports genomic stability by degrading retrotransposon RNA. Nature Communications. 2014;**5**:5276. doi:10.1038/ncomms6276

[36] Liu C, Wang H, Shang Y, Liu W, Song Z, Zhao H, et al. Autophagy is required for ectoplasmic specialization assembly in Sertoli cells. Autophagy. 2016;**12**(5):814-832. doi:10.1080/15548627.2016.1159377

[37] Gawriluk TR, Ko C, Hong XM, Christenson LK, Rucker EB. Beclin-1 deficiency in the murine ovary results in the reduction of progesterone production to promote preterm labor. Proceedings of the National Academy of Sciences of the United States of America. 2014;**111**(40):4194-4203. doi:10.1073/pnas.1409323111

[38] Terman A, Gustafsson B, Brunk UT. Autophagy, organelles and ageing. Journal of Pathology. 2007;**211**(211):134-143. doi:10.1002/path.2094

[39] Yi J, Tang XM. Functional implication of autophagy in steroid-secreting cells of the rat. The Anatomical Record. 1995;**242**(2):137-146. doi:10.1002/ar.1092420202

[40] Li WR, Chen L, Chang ZJ, Xin H, Liu T, Zhang YQ, et al. Autophagic deficiency is related to steroidogenic decline in aged rat Leydig cells. Asian Journal of Andrology. 2011;**13**(6):881-888. doi:10.1038/aja.2011.85

[41] Kroemer G, Levine B. Autophagic cell death: the story of a misnomer. Nature Reviews Molecular Cell Biology. 2008;**9**(12):1004-1010. doi:10.1038/nrm2529

[42] Madeo F, Tavernarakis N, Kroemer G. Can autophagy promote longevity?. Nature Cell Biology. 2010;**12**(9):842-846. doi:10.1038/ncb0910-842

[43] Abidi P, Zhang H, Zaidi SM, Shen WJ, Leerssucheta S, Cortez Y, et al. Oxidative stress-induced inhibition of adrenal steroidogenesis requires participation of p38 mitogen-activated protein kinase signaling pathway. Journal of Endocrinology. 2008;**198**(1):193-207. doi:10.1677/JOE-07-0570

[44] Silverstein SC, Steinman RM, Cohn ZA. Mechanisms of Endocytosis. Annual Review of Biochemistry. 2009;**78**(78):857-902. doi:10.1146/annurev.biochem.78.081307.110540

[45] Jing YI, Xue MT. The convergent point of the endocytic and autophagic pathways in leydig cells. Cell Research. 1999;**9**(4):243-53. doi:10.1038/sj.cr.7290023

[46] Nakanishi Y, Shiratsuchi A. Phagocytic removal of apoptotic spermatogenic cells by Sertoli cells: mechanisms and consequences. Biological & Pharmaceutical Bulletin. 2004;**27**(1):13. doi:10.1248/bpb.27.13

[47] Yefimova MG, Messaddeq N, Harnois T, Meunier AC, Clarhaut J, Noblanc A, et al. A chimerical phagocytosis model reveals the recruitment by Sertoli cells of autophagy for the degradation of ingested illegitimate substrates. Autophagy. 2013;**9**(5):653-66. doi:10.4161/auto.23839

[48] Rabinovitch M. Professional and non-professional phagocytes: an introduction. Trends in Cell Biology. 1995;**5**(3):85-7. doi:10.1016/S0962-8924(00)88955-2

[49] Griswold MD. The central role of Sertoli cells in spermatogenesis. Seminars in Cell & Developmental Biology. 1998;**9**(4):411-6. doi:10.1006/scdb.1998.0203

[50] Kopera IA, Bilinska B, Cheng CY, Mruk DD. Sertoli-germ cell junctions in the testis: a review of recent data. Philosophical Transactions of the Royal Society B. 2010;**365**(1546):1593-605. doi:10.1098/rstb.2009.0251

[51] Sun X, Kovacs T, Hu YJ, Yang WX. The role of actin and myosin during spermatogenesis. Molecular Biology Reports. 2011;**38**(6):3993. doi:10.1007/s11033-010-0517-0

[52] Lee NP, Cheng CY. Ectoplasmic specialization, a testis-specific cell-cell actin-based adherens junction type: is this a potential target for male contraceptive development?. Human Reproduction Update. 2004;**10**(4):349-69. doi:10.1093/humupd/dmh026

[53] Qian X, Mruk DD, Cheng YH, Tang EI, Han D, Lee WM, et al. Actin binding proteins, spermatid transport and spermiation. Seminars in Cell & Developmental Biology. 2014;**30**(6):75-85. doi:10.1016/j.semcdb.2014.04.018

[54] Wong E, Mruk D, Cy. Biology and regulation of ectoplasmic specialization, an atypical adherens junction type, in the testis. Biochimica et Biophysica Acta Biomembranes. 2008;**1778**(3):692-708. doi:10.1016/S0305-0548(99)00071-4

[55] Cheng CY, Mruk DD. The blood-testis barrier and its implications for male contraception. Pharmacological Reviews. 2012;**64**(1):16-64. doi:10.1124/pr.110.002790

[56] Hess RA, Renato dFL. Spermatogenesis and cycle of the seminiferous epithelium. Advances in Experimental Medicine & Biology. 2008;**636**(1):1-15. doi:10.1007/978-0-387-09597-4_1

[57] Vogl AW, Du M, Wang XY, Young JS. Novel clathrin/actin-based endocytic machinery associated with junction turnover in the seminiferous epithelium. Seminars in Cell & Developmental Biology. 2014;**30**(6):55-64. doi:10.1016/j.semcdb.2013.11.002

[58] Lie PPY, Mruk DD, Lee WM, Cheng CY. Cytoskeletal dynamics and spermatogenesis. Philosophical Transactions of the Royal Society B. 2010;**365**(1546):1581-92. doi:10.1098/rstb.2009.0261

[59] Upadhyay RD, Kumar AV, Ganeshan M. Tubulobulbar complex: cytoskeletal remodeling to release spermatozoa. Reproductive Biology and Endocrinology. 2012;**10**(1):27. doi:10.1186/1477-7827-10-27

[60] Tindall DJ, Mena CR, Means AR. Hormonal regulation of androgen-binding protein in hypophysectomized rats. Endocrinology. 1978;**103**(2):589-94. doi:10.1210/endo-103-2-589

[61] Karl AF, Griswold MD. Actions of insulin and vitamin A on Sertoli cells. Biochemical Journal. 1980;**186**(3):1001-3. doi:10.1042/bj1861001

[62] Aleem M, Padwal V, Choudhari J, Balasinor N, Parte P, Gill-Sharma MK. Estradiol affects androgen-binding protein expression and fertilizing ability of spermatozoa in adult male rats. Molecular & Cellular Endocrinology. 2006;**253**(1):1-13. doi:10.1016/j.mce.2006.01.014

[63] Ma Y, Yang HZ, Xu LM, Huang YR, Dai HL, Kang XN. Testosterone regulates the autophagic clearance of androgen binding protein in rat Sertoli cells. Scientific Reports. 2015;**5**:8894. doi:10.1038/srep08894

[64] Sinha Hikim AP, Swerdloff RS. Hormonal and genetic control of germ cell apoptosis in the testis. Reviews of Reproduction. 1999;**4**(1):38-47. doi:10.1530/ror.0.0040038

[65] Print CG, Loveland KL. Germ cell suicide: new insights into apoptosis during spermatogenesis. BioEssays: News and Reviews in Molecular, Cellular and Developmental Biology. 2000;**22**(5):423-30. doi:10.1002/(SICI)1521-1878(200005)22:5<423::AID-BIES4> 3.0.CO;2-0

[66] Gordy C, He YW. The crosstalk between autophagy and apoptosis: where does this lead?. Protein & Cell. 2012;**3**(1):17-27. doi:10.1007/s13238-011-1127-x

[67] Quan C, Wang C, Duan P, Huang W, Chen W, Tang S, et al. Bisphenol a induces autophagy and apoptosis concurrently involving the Akt/mTOR pathway in testes of pubertal SD rats. Environmental Toxicology. Forthcoming. doi:10.1002/tox.22339

[68] Zhang S, Niu Q, Gao H, Ma R, Lei R, Zhang C, et al. Excessive apoptosis and defective autophagy contribute to developmental testicular toxicity induced by fluoride. Environmental Pollution. 2016;**212**:97-104. doi:10.1016/j.envpol.2016.01.059

[69] Wang YJ, Yan J, Yin F, Li L, Qin Y, Meng C, et al. Role of autophagy in cadmium-induced testicular injury. Human and Experimental Toxicology. 2016;**0960327116678300**. doi:10.1177/0960327116678300

[70] Paul C, Murray AA, Spears N, Saunders PT. A single, mild, transient scrotal heat stress causes DNA damage, subfertility and impairs formation of blastocysts in mice. Reproduction. 2008;**136**(1):73-84. doi:10.1530/REP-08-0036

[71] Blackshaw AW, Massey PF. The effect of cryptorchidism on the quantitative histology, histochemistry and hydrolytic enzyme activity of the rat testis. Australian Journal of Biological Sciences. 1978;**31**(1):53. doi:10.1071/BI9780053

[72] Oberley TD, Swanlund JM, Zhang HJ, Kregel KC. Aging results in increased autophagy of mitochondria and protein nitration in rat hepatocytes following heat stress. Journal of Histochemistry & Cytochemistry. 2008;**56**(6):615-27. doi:10.1369/jhc.2008.950873

[73] Zhang M, Jiang M, Bi Y, Zhu H, Zhou Z, Sha J. Autophagy and apoptosis act as partners to induce germ cell death after heat stress in mice. PLoS One. 2012;**7**(7):e41412. doi:10.1371/journal.pone.0041412

[74] Zhang G, Liu K, Ling X, Wang Z, Zou P, Wang X, et al. DBP-induced endoplasmic reticulum stress in male germ cells causes autophagy, which has a cytoprotective role against apoptosis in vitro and in vivo. Toxicology Letters. 2016;**245**:86-98. doi:10.1016/j.toxlet.2016.01.016

[75] Liu K, Zhang G, Wang Z, Liu Y, Dong J, Dong X, et al. The protective effect of autophagy on mouse spermatocyte derived cells exposure to 1800MHz radiofrequency electromagnetic radiation. Toxicology Letters. 2014;**228**(3):216-24. doi:10.1016/j.toxlet.2014.05.004

[76] Wang Y, Zheng W, Bian X, Yuan Y, Gu J, Liu X, et al. Zearalenone induces apoptosis and cytoprotective autophagy in primary Leydig cells. Toxicology Letters. 2014;**226**(2):182-91. doi:10.1016/j.toxlet.2014.02.003

[77] Liu G, Jiang X, Zhu X, He W, Kuang Y, Ren K, et al. ROS activates JNK-mediated autophagy to counteract apoptosis in mouse mesenchymal stem cells in vitro. Acta Pharmacologica Sinica. 2015;**36**(12):1473-9. doi:10.1038/aps.2015.101

[78] Duan P, Hu C, Quan C, Yu T, Zhou W, Yuan M, et al. 4-Nonylphenol induces apoptosis, autophagy and necrosis in Sertoli cells: involvement of ROS-mediated AMPK/AKT-mTOR and JNK pathways. Toxicology. 2016;**341**:28-40. doi:10.1016/j.tox.2016.01.004

[79] Chen Y, Zhou Y, Wang X, Qian W, Han X. Microcystin-LR induces autophagy and apoptosis in rat Sertoli cells in vitro. Toxicon. 2013;**76**:84-93. doi:10.1016/j.toxicon.2013.09.005